THE WRITERS OF THE STORM

OUR JOURNEY

PATRICIA GREENE

CONTENTS

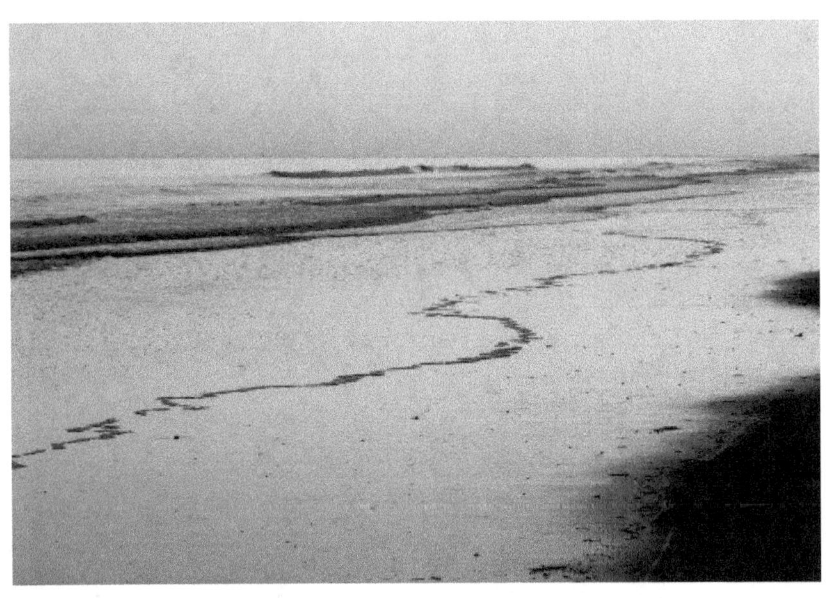

Walk with us on
"Our Journey"

Dedicated to all
That have walked this journey
And are watching over us now

"There are many whose light is so bright that it stays lit long after they are gone"

— PATTY GREENE

BREATHE

In a split second, your whole life changes. You never expected to hear those words. You never thought it could be you. But yet, here you are in that second, sitting there, your life flashing before your eyes as they tell you:

"You have Cancer"

Every cancer is different, just as every person's reaction to it is different. There are different types of cancer, different stages, and different forms of treatment. The list goes on, but the bottom line is, you have just received some of the worse news you can imagine. And at that second, all you can think of is:

"Me, I have cancer!"

Most of our emotional reactions are the same, we all think it is a death sentence. Your mind is swirling and you cannot speak. You wait for the air to return to the room, you wait for your head to stop spinning.

Then the battle begins.

The following stories are from amazing people, who heard those words. After they pulled themselves together, they did the only thing they knew how to do.

Fight back!

It is hard to fight such an unseen enemy, it is hard to try to put a face to it, and it is hard to be strong. We all come from different lifestyles it doesn't matter who you are. But one thing we all know for sure is that there is something deep inside that tells us we cannot give up and we decide to give it all we have.

Most of these stories touch home with me. I have known some of these people as they walked through their battle. I have watched as this beast has torn through families. I have also seen the amazing strength that it takes to get up every day and fight for yourself, and I have witnessed the fight that we take on for our loved ones.

Cancer changes everything. It changes your perspective on life, it gives you clarity on what is important. For some of us, it reconnects us to God or higher purpose and mends broken ties. It is hard not to fall into that "Why me" and become a victim, or to be angry. I think most of us give in to it for a little while.

I would like you to take the time and absorb all of these amazing stories from the people who have taken the time to share with you. They have opened up their hearts and souls to give hope, and to inspire us all.

When the going gets tough, the tough get going!

INTRODUCTION

BY PATRICIA GREENE

It's kind of funny when I think about it. I always wanted to write a book. I loved to write poetry, I loved to write short stories, and I loved to make up stories with my children when they were little. We used to play that game where one person would say a sentence and then the next person would have to come up with the next line. We would laugh at the silly things that each one of us would come up with. I never thought I would ever be able to put a book together, even though I know I have an amazing story to tell about my life. However, dropping out of school in the 10th grade really hurt my self-confidence, and I didn't think I was smart enough to ever write my book. Even after I got my GED and passed it with flying colors, went to college and did really well, I still didn't think I was "good enough – smart enough" to ever pull it off.

I was wrong. When you are passionate about something and you really truly care, you can find a way, and I did! My first book was about the struggles with families and addiction. It came from something that has touched my life. My oldest child, Daniel, passed from an overdose. He had struggled for 22 years with Substance Abuse Disorder. That monster took my son away from us long before he died. I would get glimpses of him from time to time, but when he was in the throes of addiction, he was a different person. My son was a kind, loving person who cared so much about family and friends. His death was so hard on all of us. And once again we learned the lesson of how short life can be. This wasn't the first time I had tragedy happen in my life.

My second book was also about struggles with addiction, but these stories were different. I broke it into 3 parts, 1st part was the tragic loss of loved ones, the 2nd part was stories about recovery. These brave souls shared their stories about their journey to addiction and then from addiction. If you have young teenagers, I suggest you read these stories. The 3rd part is about people who deal with this all the time, the people who answer the call when a loved one is in trouble or has passed. In addition, stories from people who help fight for people suffering, knowing their battles. Both of my books are available on Amazon. I will put a link to them at the end of this book.

Now, I have started my own book about me, it is still a work in progress. I have been working on it for a very long time but now it is finally starting to take shape. I hope to finish it by the end of 2024.

That brings me to this one. "The Writers of The Storm" The storm of course being cancer. The cover shows the ocean so calm and peaceful, not knowing what can be brewing underneath.. Just like cancer, we can look fine on the outside while a storm is going on inside. Many of these stories in this book refer to the storm. I think it was only fitting to name the book after the Writers of The Storm.

I am a breast cancer survivor, so cancer has touched me and my family. It has made me aware of how precious life is and how everything can change in a nanosecond. It has shown me both the ugly side of it and the beautiful side of it. I may never understand the whys of it, but I know that we as humans will not give up without a fight.

Because of the breast cancer, I found this amazing group of women a few years after my diagnosis in 2010. I would like to introduce my Braveheart sisters. This group was founded by some pretty amazing people. (I will also supply a link to their website and Facebook page.) These women get together 3 or 4 times a year at "camp". It sounded amazing, but I never felt like I was able to go because I was raising my granddaughter and married, my obligations never allowed me. That however changed in the year 2023, she was old enough to be on her own and I was recently divorced from a 20-year marriage. I was broken in many ways and I felt it was time to do something for myself, so I went to meet these amazing women at camp!

My first camp was at Shelter Island NY. I was so excited yet also a little nervous. I didn't know what to expect, those old doubts, "Am I going to fit in? Am I going to be the outsider? Am I going to like it? What if I can't sleep? (I suffer from insomnia) The list went on and on. I wanted to go so badly, yet I think I was trying to talk myself out of it. I am happy to say, that those negative thoughts did not win and I went to camp.

I was met with open arms, big smiles, and "glad you finally made it!" I was in! I felt so much love. The bus trip to shelter island was wonderful, all of us talking about our life in general. Some of us took a snooze along the way, others were quietly thinking. Many were laughing. It was really so amazing.

Then we got to Shelter Island, YEE HAW.. wow! I was blown away. It was beautiful and there were more women, a whole other bus full, and others driving in! I felt this deep comfort in my stomach; I felt love…

That was only the beginning. The 4 days flew by with so many things to do, awesome meals and time to share and talk to others. We played silly games that made us laugh so hard we cried. We were pampered and cared for. I thought, so THIS is what I have been missing all this time!

For me, it was also a time to reflect and heal from the past few years. It was time for me to just let it all go and live in the moment. My heart was so full of gratitude. All of these amazing women sharing their journey with each other, but doing so in way you would never expect. It wasn't self-pity and it wasn't a challenge of whose journey was worst. If was support, love, acceptance. They also had full hearts of gratitude.

I came home with the idea of another book. I put it on the back burner for a while, because I had to think about what I wanted to do and how I wanted to do it. I just went on with my daily hectic routine.

In October 2023, I went to the next camp at Double H in New York. This trip changed me. I did not only bond with a whole bunch of new people, I bonded with myself.

However, my AHA moment was one afternoon I was sitting alone at my table in the cafeteria just watching and listening to everyone chatting and laughing. Then all of a sudden I could not hear them anymore, I could feel them. The energy that each one of these amazing women were releasing and putting into each other. I could feel the tears roll down my cheek. I knew I was experiencing something for which there was no human explanation. In the midst of all of that, I also knew right then that their stories and energy needed to be shared. There were a few that seem to actually stand out more than others, like an inner light came on in them and they were beaming. I don't know how much time went by, but I knew what I wanted to do. I just didn't know if they were willing.

Cancer is something that many of us fear. We all see the nasty side of it. I have also seen the other side of it. I have seen communities come together to support a family when a loved one has been diagnosed with it. I have seen the most amazing display of love for one another who is suffering. I have seen what the spirit of love can do.

For those whose journey was over, I was blessed to have known them; they were a gift to me. And they will forever hold the highest place of love in my heart. They are missed greatly, but they live on in all of us. They keep us strong and fuel us with the desire to make a difference.

I hope you enjoy these stories and understand what courage it took for these people to write about their journey. I know a lot of tears were shed remembering as they walked down memory lane.

I asked a good friend of mine who works at Hahne Cancer Clinic in Dubois, Pa to start the book off with her story. She is an amazing person and I am so grateful to call her my friend. Jean Levin, Advanced Oncology Certified Nurse Practitioner.

WHAT DO YOU WANT TO BE WHEN YOU GROW UP?

BY JEAN LEVIN

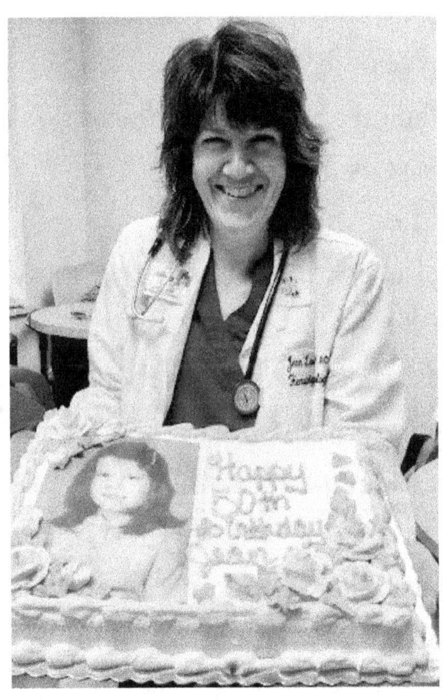

I was 17 years old sitting in the guidance counselor's class trying to answer this very question. How was I supposed to know what I wanted to do? I never really had any plans, I never dreamed of being an astronaut or a cowgirl; all I wanted to do was survive high school. Then I was facing graduation into real life; out came the aptitude test. Some of the questions I remember answering on this test included:

1. *Do you want to wear a uniform?* Answer: how do I know? I'm in a public school.
2. *Do you like people?* Answer (at that time) yes I guess I like people.
3. *Would you want to help other people?* Answer: I suppose I could help people.
4. *Do you like to work on vehicles?* Answer: Is that what a screwdriver is used for?

Without much thought, I decided to follow my four older sisters into the nursing profession. (I always joked that my smart older sister became the teacher). Anyway, four years later after many late nights, tears, fears faced, and only one failing grade, I graduated from Indiana State University with a Bachelor's of Science in Nursing (BSN). The year was 1988 and BSN-prepared nurses were not very common in the DuBois hospital where I started my nursing career. I can remember one of the physicians asking me where I went to school and his reply after I told him was "oh you are one of those nurses." My immediate thought was (well let's keep this

PG) what does that mean? What does "those nurses" mean? A woman with a college degree? Yes, I am a woman with a college degree and I will show you just how great a nurse I will become. So, with much determination, I learned and mentored with the best "seasoned" nurses I could find; and excellent nurses they were! I also volunteered to round with the doctors (when most nurses didn't have the time to spare to go with the doctors) and asked many questions. The best physicians would share their stories and teach me all they could: a mostly enjoyable experience. I grew in knowledge and experience.

The unit I was assigned was the inpatient oncology floor, I worked the 3 to 11 pm shift (yes there was a day many moons ago that nurses worked an 8 hour shift) that is where I got to first experience caring for cancer patients.

As some of you may know, the Hahne Cancer Center was completed in 1988 as the vision of one of the excellent physicians of the DuBois hospital. He saw a great need for our community and brought the vision of a cancer center to the region. No longer did patients need to travel hours away to receive their cancer care, it was now available in our back yard. I still remember going to Geisinger medical center in the late 1970's with my father to visit my uncle as he was treated for head and neck cancer and what a toll it took on my family.

When the cancer center patients needed inpatient chemo-therapy or care due to their illnesses, they were admitted to my unit. I absolutely loved caring for these patients. They were the most gracious people I ever met. From saying "thank you" (when they got a popsicle) and saying "God bless you" just because you showed up to work, it was nice to be treated with respect and as a human!

I set my sights on getting hired into the outpatient unit. I studied everything I could and took a class at Fox Chase Cancer Center where I spent a week taking their Oncology Nursing Society (ONS) chemotherapy course. I learned about oncologic emergencies, classes of chemotherapy agents, and then did "hands on" where I got to give the treatments to patients. I then became "OCN" certified (Oncology certified nurse), one of the first on the inpatient unit.

As the cancer center grew, so did the need for additional nurses, so when a full-time job came up in late 1992, I jumped on it! I remember dressing up for the interview. Following all my hard work, I landed the job and can still remember going home and telling my husband "I will never have to work another Christmas again;" what little did I know!

I started my career at the cancer center in early 1993. At that time, the nurses did all the jobs. We scheduled appointments, labs, and imaging. Got insurance authorizations for medications, doctor visits, and scans. We roomed the patients, took vital signs, assisted the doctors with exams and bone marrows, we also made the calendars for patients so they would remember their treatment dates. But the number one job was to give the chemotherapy. We had 6 chairs and 2 beds in our little center. Two nurses would draw the labs, start the IV's, go mix the chemotherapy and then administer it; all the while assessing and educating our patients on the side effects and management of those treatments. We even gave blood transfusions in our little space. We were busy, there was always something to do and learn, but I still felt like I could do more. I continued to feel like I didn't know what my purpose in life was about. One day I was approached by my friend and colleague about a program that he wanted me to do called "nurse practitioner." I asked, "what is that?" And he said, "don't worry about it, just do it!" The program was at the University of Pittsburgh and they had a sub-specialty in oncology. He gave me the contact number, so I called. The secretary was extremely pleasant and said "Great! Classes start tomorrow." So that night I sat down with my husband and talked about this program. He was totally on board with it and supported my decision. My huge concern was that we had 3 young daughters at home and he said, "I will raise the girls."

The next day, I was sitting in a classroom at the Johnstown campus of Pitt in a class called pathophysiology (at that time I couldn't even pronounce the word let alone know what the heck it was). After the class finished, I looked around the room, thinking to myself "what the hell are you doing here?" and I locked eyes with another girl who had the exact same expression on her face. The next week, we both showed up (me with a tape recorder, it was 1997) and her with a little smirk on her face because half of the class did not return. The second class turned out to be much better and we all figured out that the professor was "weeding out" the quitters with the first lesson. It turns out that the girl I locked eyes with became one of my best friends through the program and together we graduated 3 years later summa cum laude both specializing in oncology. She started in Johnstown and I in DuBois and we both continue to work at our original places of employment.

I graduated on 4/30/2000, my oldest daughter's birthday, and started as a nurse practitioner on 5/1/2000. I can tell you it was one of the hardest jobs I have ever done. I cried every single night for the first 6 months because I was terrified I would make a mistake and hurt a patient. My respect for doctors skyrocketed and eventually the crying stopped. I can still remember standing outside an exam room door, taking a deep breath, sticking up my chin and thinking you can do this! So much to know, so much to learn, but with kindness and respect you can conquer your fears. The doctors were amazing, the staff supportive, but the best part about the new job was the patients. They accepted me with open arms and I grew to love them all. I got the opportunity to see things from a different perspective. I was now helping them make treatment decisions and making sure they got the best care possible, whether that was at our facility or referring them to a tertiary care center. I felt that my true calling may have been answered.

Almost 24 years later, I am still doing what I love. My work with the patients is why I show up every day. The patients. They are what inspire me to be the best at my job. The patients. The reason I became a nurse. The patients. The reason I became a nurse practitioner. The patients. The career path I chose at the age of 17.

I could have sat here and told you all the stories about my patients but those are their stories to tell. I am their health-care provider, I am their sounding board, I am their confidant, and lots of times I am their friend. I cannot tell you what it is like to go through a cancer diagnosis, I have not gone down that path yet in my life. But I can tell you what it is like to care for a loved one with cancer, that path I have been down many times with family member and now every day with my patients.

I can only tell you that I love what I do and I am thankful I got the opportunity to do this life work. To my patients: thank you for letting me serve you. To my patients: thank you for teaching me humility. To my patients: thank you for teaching me love. To my patients: thank you for allowing me to be a part of your life.

To those I have lost, to those I have helped cure, to those I have not met yet, thank you.

So what do I want to be when I grow up? Unemployed! I want cancer to be a thing of the past (like 8-hour shifts for nurses). I want to sit on a mountain, drinking coffee with my family, petting my dogs, watching the sunrise and thankful I no longer have a job.

But maybe, just maybe I will get that screwdriver and start working on my car.

Jean Levin CRNP, MSN, AOCNP

Yes, I still have my certification, but it is now Advanced oncology certified nurse practitioner and I ended up caring for that doctor who made the comment about "those nurses" (he became my patient). Turns out he was a great person and I thank him for pushing me to be the best I could be!

Thank You.

2

LIVING LIFE WITH MEDICAL TRAUMA

BY JEANNIE

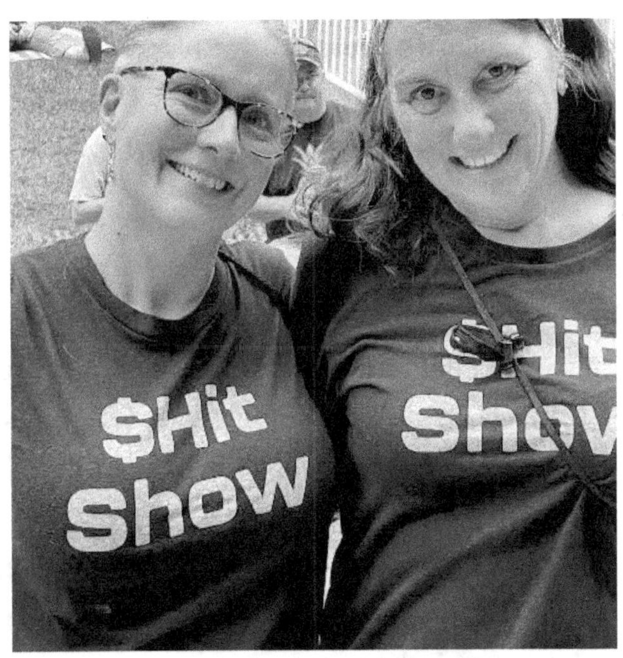

My story started over fifty years ago when I was born with a congenital kidney disease. I was undiagnosed and very sick from birth to three years old. I spent most of my early life in and out of hospitals. At the age of three, I had three major abdominal surgeries in three weeks. I had a nephrectomy and total reconstruction of my kidney system. By age five, I began to thrive and started school with my childhood peers. Throughout my childhood and into my adult life, I lived with this disease.

Fast forward to age 45, in 2012, I was informed that I would have to have a kidney transplant or dialysis as my kidney was failing. In 2012, one of my best friends donated one of her kidneys to me. A successful transplant gave me my life back. I felt ten years younger, not realizing how sick I was when in post-op recovery; I could have done cartwheels!

One year later (2013), I had my routine mammogram. I was called back for more films and a week after, a mammo-assisted biopsy. During this barbaric biopsy, with my face stuffed up against the plexiglass and hearing this drilling in my ear, there was a surreal moment whereby my surgeon looked at me and said, "You can rest your head on my shoulder, OK?" I calmly said, "OK," and passed out cold. When I awoke, numerous blue-scrubbed staff with bright eyes stood over me. My colleagues and long-time friends were caring for me instead of me caring for them.

About a week later, while just arriving to work at the hospital for night supervision, I was informed by a phone call by my surgeon that I had breast cancer. I will never forget that call. I sat in the office chair for 45 minutes; I couldn't move. I was frozen in time. I cried a little but mostly just sat there in shock.

A week after, I had a lumpectomy and thirty-five radiation treatments over seven weeks. My surgeon suggested a bilateral mastectomy, much like Angelina Jolie. At this point in breast cancer care, it was the push to have them removed; EVERYONE was doing it! I told my surgeon there was no way I could handle another major surgery as I was still healing from the kidney transplant.

Thereafter, denial was my protective shield. I went to work at night, did radiation treatment in the mornings, and told no one what was happening. Easy right? I was so wrong. I "dealt" with it alone without any support because I felt like my consistent medical issues were a burden on my family, friends, and work. I did not take the advice I gave patients every day.

Life went on, and I did my due diligence with mammograms/ultrasounds every six months, with scanxiety for a week prior every single time. After five years - ALL CLEAR! But was I?

Fast forward to 2020, the global pandemic and hell embarked upon us all. Being immunocompromised, I was super cautious. I followed the CDC guidelines bestowed on us and received my vaccines as recommended for compromised patients. Believe it or not, I did not get COVID during this time. That came later.......

In 2021, the post-COVID surge lifted. I went on vacation with my sister-in-law, and on return, our flights were canceled and rescheduled on a different route. On the 3rd of July, the airline overnighted us in Charlotte, N.C. On the 4th of July morning, we entered the lobby to get the shuttle back to the airport. Before the shuttle's arrival, I went to the lobby restroom and did not return. My sister found me on the bathroom floor unresponsive, lying half in the stall and half out, in all my glory, pants to my knees. Emergency services were activated and quickly arrived (there was a marathon in the city nearby). EMS resuscitated and took me to Atrium Health, bypassing Duke and another major medical center. Atrium Health has the best neurosurgical department in the country, per Sam, the paramedic. My Jane Doe name was "Pineapple." The emergency physician and staff activated the "Code Stroke" call, and after the brain CT, they determined that I had a ruptured brain aneurysm. I was quickly sedated, intubated, and put on life support—two brain surgeries in twenty-four hours. The whiteboard in my patient room stated, "I am a nurse," which was code for all staff to know. Needless to say, I was not a good patient. On day four (4), I regained active consciousness and remembered very little. My husband, daughter, and sister-in-law were at my bedside. I lived five minutes at a time with a cerebral spinal fluid

(CSF) tube in my skull. By week three in the neuro ICU, I was strong enough to face the 16-hour ride in the car home. Due to fatigue and terrible headaches, it took us three days to get home. I was never so happy to be home.

After that, six months of outpatient occupational and physical therapy. This recovery was the hardest yet. I had to learn to walk (without falling), whole body strengthening, and relearn simple tasks—slow motion healing. I am forever grateful that the timing was impeccable at every turn, and I had a fantastic support system. I went back to work on the 3rd of January, 2022. I slowly regained my work life, re-engaged in my social life, and exercised. I was determined to return to my former state of physical and mental health. All good, right? Enough?? Not a chance......

On the 25th of April, I had my annual mammogram/ultrasound, and guess what? I was called back for more films and then a mammogram-assisted biopsy of the left breast. No, this test hadn't changed in eight years! It's still a barbaric masculine tale top drill! This time, I did not pass out because I screamed as loud as I could with every injection. The absolute most painful thing in the world of healthcare procedures! My surgeon said, "I believe you have an intolerance to lidocaine with epinephrine." YOU THINK?????? My girlfriend (nurse) insisted on driving me, and thank goodness she did! From the waiting area, she could hear someone screaming, never thinking it was me! I shook in shock for an hour afterward. I was unable to drive home. My gut instinct was telling me that this is not good. These results were going to be positive. My gut is always right.

On the 29th of April, I was at work (second job) at the community college where I teach during office hours. I received a phone call from my primary care doctor. He was excitable and rambling about all the changes we would have to make to my immunosuppression drugs and obtain the blood work for genetic testing. I interrupted him and asked him what was going on. He questioned me, "You don't know?" I said, "Don't know what? Better start telling me now." He received the results before my surgeon could tell me. She was consulting with my oncologist. This time, I called my best friend; I immediately went to her house and fell apart in the driveway in her arms.

A different breast cancer-Aggressive Ductal Invasive Carcinoma (DIC) of the breast, was diagnosed. "Very ominous; we need to work fast........"

Due to our large geographic area, my care was split between two aggressively competitive small-town rural community hospitals; my surgeon worked at one, and the cancer treatment/primary care doctor at the other. I spent five weeks trying to navigate my cancer care. Nurse navigators were eliminated years prior, and I was caught in the middle. Who gets the patient? It was baffling to me that I was not told where to go. It was ASSUMED I would stay local. No, not this time. I wanted to ensure that I wasn't going to have a nipple on my forehead! Continually, I was told where NOT to go. I quickly realized I needed to step up and advocate for myself as I would for any of my patients. Use my resources/tools, call in my favors, and be aggressive.

Finally, I was referred to Memorial Sloan Kettering (MSK) by my primary care physician (my lifesaver and calvery). By the 1st of June, I had a plan for a bilateral mastectomy. I was 99% sure I was going to go aesthetic all-flat. My plastic surgeon at MSK convinced me to have reconstruction-breast implants. "You are young; they will be perky; silicone implants after tissue expanders," she said. I should have gone with my gut instinct! Always listen to your gut!

I will say that MSK was fantastic. The bilateral mastectomy was conducted on the 1st of July, 2022. I was discharged home the next day to begin yet another healing. My best friend set her van up for the seven-hour trip home from NYC.

Then, the longest and worst recovery yet......

Because of the previous DCIS with radiation, the breast tissue on the right chest would not heal, thus rendering the right tissue expander challenging to fill. From day one post-op, I suffered from daily pain, multiple seromas, and bizarre skin rashes. Within the first month of recovery, the pain was increasingly horrific. My right breast was red, hot, and spongy. Something was wrong! Again, I couldn't get any help. My surgeon was out of town. I needed a doctor's order to have an ultrasound. The local emergency room would not touch it because the surgeon was out of the area. "You need to go back to that surgeon." WHAT???? So, off to NYC, we went. My plastic surgeon's nurse pulled 100 ccs of yellow serous drainage off the right side—a seroma. The relief was instant but short-lived.

Within 24 hours, the seroma was back, and I was home. I continued to suffer for a few days, praying that it would just go away. The anxiety this caused was overpowering. I was telling my nurse friend about the situation. I told her that if I had a needle, syringe, and tubing, I would have her draw it off. She then informed me that Tractor Supply has what we need. I told her I would be there in twenty minutes. Off to tractor supply, I went, where I picked up syringes and (bovine) needles! I then went to her house, where we set up her bed as a procedure area and drew more fluid off. It drained for hours afterward.

A couple of weeks later, it had to be drained again. We were at a camp on the St. Lawrence River and used the kitchen center counter as a procedure table this time. My friends got me through these difficult six months.

In late August, I met with my surgeon for a final fill. Due to the skin being red, taunt, and shiny, she was reluctant to fill the right side and indicated she wanted me to see the plastic surgeon in NYC.

Between this visit and the NYC plastics appointment, I developed a rash across my abdomen - it looked like shingles but wasn't. At the same time, I developed an abrasion (dime-sized) at 9 o'clock on the right breast. It looked like a scrape. It then became a scab and sloughed off. My plastic surgeon took one look at it and informed me that we could not do the implant on that side. She told me of the option to do a latissimus dorsi flap (skin graph) off my back or go all-flat. I was informed that I had time to "think" about it. The expanders can stay in for extended periods (years), so I was to let her know when I was ready to do what I decided. Ultimately, I decided to go aesthetic all-flat, in May 2023.

During this, I was caring for my elderly 92-year-old mother, who was exhibiting signs of dementia, caught shingles, and needed 24-hour care. I had to place her in an elder home. This was heartbreaking and stressful at the same time.

While caring for her at the elder home, I slept on a cot beside her bed. She was under hospice care now, having had three strokes. During Thanksgiving week, she deteriorated to total care. I slept there nightly and assisted with her care. On day three, I woke at 4:30 in the morning to find my nightshirt soaked. An infectious smell overpowered me. I went directly to the bathroom mirror to see a gaping hole (the size of a quarter) in my right chest. Black center-oozing infection. I had some pain, but because nerves are severed during mastectomies, I was numb. Just my normal daily pain.....

I frantically texted and phoned my surgeon, cancer treatment center, and my primary care. I went to the Emergency Room, and I was told that I had a significant infection and the expander needed to come out NOW. I was given IV Vancomycin and pain medication. I was offered to have the expander out there, even though, admittedly, the surgeon had never done this. "No" was the answer. I needed to be with my mom until she passed. What I needed was antibiotics to bridge me until she passed and only then would I go to NYC for bilateral explant surgery, removing it all.

My mother died on the 1st of December, 2022, at 1:30 in the morning in my arms. I was on the road by 6:00 am, headed to NYC for emergency surgery. Sleep-deprived and grief-stricken, I rode the train to NYC with my friend and my husband and wrote my mom's obituary.

The MSK surgery team held me up and cried with me. They walked me to the operating room suite and helped me onto the table. My plastic surgeon gave me condolences with tears in her eyes, and I begged them to put me to sleep.........

Immediately upon the completion of this surgery and removal of the tissue expanders, I felt more myself than I had in six months. The rash went completely away; my pain reduced significantly. I healed and recovered from this bilateral explant surgery in less than three weeks.

I still cannot fathom the magnitude of what my body and mind have endured. My mom would tell me- to write the book. I would tell her, " I don't know who would believe it."

LESSONS LEARNED:

1. Be an advocate for yourself!
2. Know there are so many decisions, and they are hard to make.
3. Have a notebook- write it all down chronologically, and include the names of the healthcare team!
4. Don't do what I did- seek medical care (not at Tractor Supply)!
5. Ask questions and know your options. You can refuse if you feel the plan is not for you, and you can obtain a second or third opinion.
6. Be loud and proud!
7. Take someone with you, and this might not be your spouse. This person needs to know intimate details about your history. You may not be able to comprehend what is being said. This person is your second voice and will remember things you don't.
8. You are the patient, and now all revolves around YOU!

3

THE DAY THE EARTH FELL OFF ITS AXIS

BY CHERYL CLARK

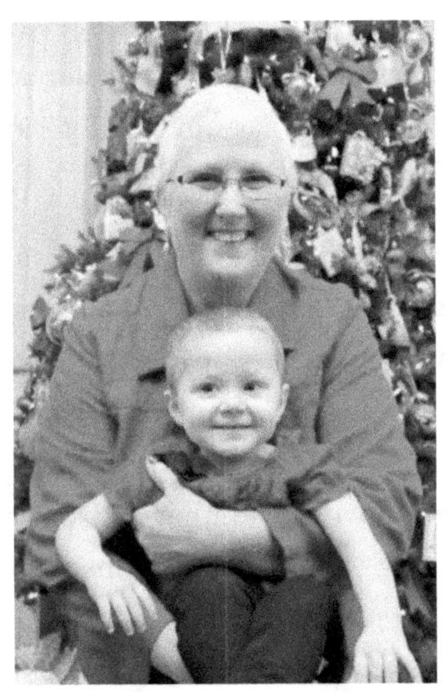

My cancer journey began in January 2013. I had put off my yearly mammogram for 14 months and when I finally got around to getting it done, I received a call from the nurse at the medical imaging facility afterward asking me to return for more imaging and to bring a family member with me. The nurse on the phone said, "That way if you receive bad news you have someone with you for support and if you receive good news you have someone to celebrate with." Both of my adult daughters were with me when I received the news that I had stage 0, "intraductal carcinoma in situ" breast cancer. It was a devastating moment that none of us will ever forget. The "good news" was that it was stage zero and had not spread outside of the milk ducts in my breast. It was contained but I really had no idea what that meant, what any of it meant. We had no family history of breast cancer.

I called my gynecologist, the doctor who had ordered my mammogram and who had delivered all three of my grand-children. I was frantic to find out my next steps. I was flailing about with no idea about what to do, I couldn't even think straight. I heard nothing back, in fact ten years later I have never heard a word from her or from her office. I felt abandoned at one of the worst moments of my life and I was terrified. I contacted the imaging facility and spoke with the radiologist who had diagnosed my breast cancer. She was so kind to me and referred me to a breast surgeon and recom-mended an Oncology-Hematology practice to call.

After meeting with the surgeon, I decided to have a lumpectomy in February 2013 and was developing a treatment plan with my oncologist for post surgery. However, after the pathology report came back I received the news that more cancer was found and it was outside of the milk duct. The tumor was still small but, now my cancer was stage one, ER+ HER2neu+ breast cancer. I was alone when I received this news and discovered why, in fact, the medical imaging facility wanted you to bring someone with you. I hadn't expected bad news after my lumpectomy so went on my own to the follow up appointment. After getting the news that my cancer was worse than initially diagnosed, I remember driving from my appointment to meet my mom and sister at my mom's doctor's office so I wouldn't be alone. I was on auto pilot and I was in such shock that I drove to the wrong place. That is why you don't go alone, you go into shock and really need someone with you to help you get your bearings.

I met with my surgeon again and opted for a second lumpectomy in March 2013 hoping I wasn't being a fool for not having a mastectomy instead. The pathology report after my second surgery showed clean margins, indicating that my surgeon had gotten all of the cancer and that there wasn't any spread to my lymph nodes. This was fabulous news and after I healed from the lumpectomy, I would be able to begin my treatment plan with my oncologist. I took my entire family out for dinner that Friday night to celebrate the ecstatic news. What a relief!

Two days later, on Sunday, March 24, 2013 the world stopped moving for a moment, and then literally came off its axis, spinning uncontrollably into space. That was the day when my youngest daughter called me from the emergency room at Albany Medical Center to tell me to get there immediately, that they found a mass in my youngest granddaughter's abdomen. Kennedy was 17 months old. On Valentine's Day 2013 my son in law and I felt something funny on the side of her tummy but she didn't complain when we pressed on it so it didn't seem urgent enough to run to the emergency room, which is where my panicky daughter wanted to go. In hindsight, that is exactly where we should have gone! Instead, we were practical and the next day took her to the pediatrician's office and saw the doctor on call. That doctor misdiagnosed the mass as a "floating rib" stating it was nothing to worry about. That sounded very odd but what did we know? Again, in hindsight we wish the doctor had said, "I'm pretty sure it is a floating rib but let's send her for an X-ray to be certain." So another month passed and when Kennedy couldn't keep food down, she was taken to Albany Medical Center and officially diagnosed.

When I arrived at the emergency room, it was pure bedlam in the waiting area but when I checked in at the desk I was immediately rushed past the other people waiting, into a private room in the back where my family waited. That seemed odd to me but I was impressed with their expediency. Then, I became so confused when I was introduced to a social worker who was there with Kennedy, my daughter

Lauren, her husband Nate, and Kennedy's paternal grandmother Ann, all sequestered inside this private room. Before I had a chance to receive any information or ask any questions, a doctor came into the room. Her name was Dr. N and she was a somewhat intimidating figure both in her size and demeanor. It turns out that Dr. N was a pediatric oncologist, and an angel. I was so confused in that moment, I asked, "Why was an oncologist necessary, it was just a mass. They could remove it and all would be okay, right?" Then my daughter turned to me and said, "No mom, Kennedy has cancer, the mass is cancer." That is the moment that the earth fell off its axis. I had just received clean margins and had been celebrating and two days later ALL of our lives were forever changed. Kennedy had stage 4 Hepatoblastoma, a childhood liver cancer that babies are born with. It manifests itself usually around 18 months of age. Kennedy's cancer had metastasized to her lungs, onto her liver, and to her gall bladder. The tumor was the size of a football in her tiny body and was inoperable if they couldn't shrink it down.

This is where our cancer journeys converge and something amazing happened to me. All the terror I had felt regarding my cancer diagnosis disappeared. I was praying so hard for God to please take me, not Kennedy, and I meant it to my very soul. It wasn't about me anymore, and that little, precious child showed me how to go through treatment with grace, without complaint, and how to be fearless. I began my course of treatment with two types of chemo and a year of Herceptin infusions. This was followed by radiation and then ten years of Anastrazole (Arimidex). Kennedy began chemo the night she was diagnosed. The protocol for her chemo hadn't changed in fifty years yes, fifty years! It was literally watered down adult chemo. Yet, I received the latest in research for what chemo should be given for my specific cancer, a smart drug that only attacked cancer cells and left the healthy cells alone, and ten years of a drug to keep my cancer away.

Thankfully, Kennedy's tumor responded to the intense chemo she was given and the tumor began to shrink. Most of her life was spent in the pediatric unit at Albany Med and her parents either shared a recliner each night or one slept on the floor while the other slept in the chair. The room was a double so other cancer kid families slept on the other side of the curtain with their child. It was crazy but I rarely heard them complain. My oldest daughter and her husband took care of Lauren and Nate's oldest child who was only 3-1/2 at the time. This was a traumatic time for everyone in my family. My daughter and son in law couldn't work during this time and it was a financial hardship for them in addition to the emotional toll.

Once the tumor shrank to a size where they could operate safely, Kennedy had surgery to remove 60% of her liver and her gall bladder. The pediatric surgeon and the adult liver surgeon he would be operating with had difficulty coming up with a surgery date that would work for both of them. Dr. Ganey, another angel doctor, had vacation plans with his family in the Outer Banks. After a sleepless night where he thought about Kennedy and then looked at his own healthy children, he sent his family on vacation and stayed behind to perform the surgery plus three days to make sure she was okay post-op before rejoining them. He told me that he just couldn't leave in good conscience with what our family was going through. He now practices surgery in Africa with Doctors Without Borders, a truly special human being! It is a good thing he stayed the extra days because he had nicked a bile duct during surgery and had to remove 200 staples to find the leak and repair it wearing those binoculars doctors wear for that type of almost microscopic surgery. Kennedy had an incision that was 50% of her body so to find the leak must have been incredibly challenging.

After Kennedy healed enough to move out of the PICU and onto the pediatric floor, I took her to the Ronald MacDonald room to play one day. I remember that I was experiencing some neuropathy from chemo and was limping a little but she had neuropathy way worse than mine and was so driven by the thought of playing that she nearly ran down the hall, limping noticeably while holding the walls for support. Meanwhile, I was having trouble keeping up while wheeling her IV pole behind her along the way. I never paid any attention to my neuropathy after that.

Basically, Kennedy never knew that this wasn't normal life for every other toddler in the world and did not have any frame of reference to complain about much in her life. Oh I know there were times when chemo made her so sick and the Zofran didn't help. Her parents got the brunt of all that but they never complained. After Kennedy's successful surgery, my daughter said to me, "Kennedy has a 60% chance of recurrence after her treatment is over." I immediately said, "Yeah, but she has a 40% chance that she won't have a recurrence and that is where she is going to fall!" Honestly. I couldn't bear the thought of my daughter losing her little girl and me having to pick up the pieces of her shattered life. I prayed so hard for God to please take me instead! I had a 2% chance of recurrence.

At this point in our journeys, I was getting ready for radiation to start and Kennedy was getting ready to begin even more intense chemo than she had before her liver resection, including the red devil (Doxorubicin). She had a 100% chance of losing some or all of her hearing from the Cisplatin she had to take. It didn't matter, the only thing that mattered at this point was getting rid of the cancer on her lungs. Miracles do happen and not only did the spots on her lungs completely disappear but she beat 100% odds and lost none of her hearing! By late September 2013 both Kennedy and I were NED (no evidence of disease) and we were both deemed cancer free, our hair was beginning to come back in too!

Sadly, Dr. Nepo passed away from cancer a number of years ago. The fabulous doctor who scared many of the Residents and others at Albany Med with her bullish ways was gone.

She had literally pushed her way into the operating room with Kennedy to perform her biopsy, making adult patients with less urgent surgeries wait to go under the knife. If you ever had surgery that was delayed, now you know why. Dr. N then hand carried a small mountain of samples directly from the operating room to the pathologist and sat next to him throughout the process of testing them. I know, I was there when she came out to tell us curtly that "Kennedy was in recovery doing fine but that, as we can see (showing the small mountain of samples), she needed to get the samples to pathology to test everything." She was all business until her little patients were well and then she softened, and you knew that every child in her care was treated as her child, the child she never had but loved just the same.

Fast forward to 2023 and both Kennedy and I are still cancer free and healthy. She has been back once a year for check ups at the Melody Center for Childhood Cancer while I am still going every six months to see my oncologist. I do have PTSD from all that happened but manage it pretty well most of the time. I retired five years ago and travel a lot, I really have a great life! My daughter Lauren ended up becoming a Pediatric Oncology nurse at Albany Med after the dust settled in her life. She still works as a nurse but in a school for severely handicapped students that require tube feedings and other critical care. She also works per diem at Albany Med as a pediatric nurse. I think that giving back is her therapy.

Kennedy is on the high honor roll in 7th grade while taking honors math and science classes. She is on the swim team at school and dances on 7 different competitive dance teams outside of school. She has no known side effects from her cancer. Her liver has grown in size to make up for the 60% she lost, although it has grown in the wrong direction. It functions perfectly so no one is concerned. I think that she is destined to do great things, maybe even find a cure for childhood cancer. She has no memories of her cancer journey and isn't defined by it in any way. She is just a happy, normal kid! I learned so much from her along our journey together, I am so grateful, each and every day!

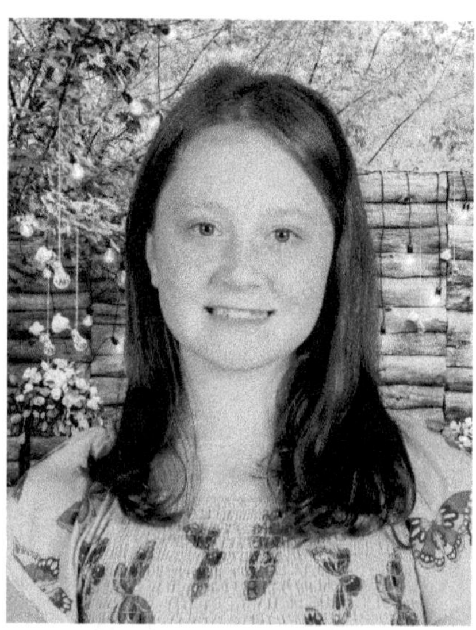

Kennedy 2023

4

IT WAS A BEAUTIFUL MEMORIAL DAY WEEKEND

BY CYNDILOU

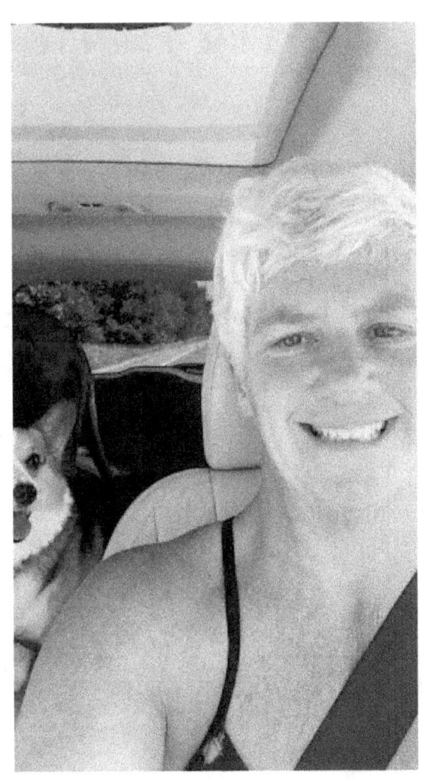

My house was clean and my yard work done. I did an 18 mile bike ride for exercise, and I was able to zip up and down all the hills.   I had recently lost over 128lbs over the course of almost 2 years, and I was determined to keep working on it.

After my bike ride I had a hard time catching my breath. I couldn't fully expand to get a deep breath. So I told my ex I was going to ER to make sure it wasn't a Pulmonary Embolism, which was a risk due to some of the more physical activities I engaged in. I thought I maybe dislodged a clot from my legs. I went to local ER where I worked as an RN. My labs were perfect and there was no sign of an embolism. However, there was a finding of atelectasis which is "lazy lung."

I questioned that immediately because I should not have it due to the intense bike ride I just took. I told the doctor that I had vomited while driving on the highway, then immediately felt great. Based on this, the doctor ordered an ultrasound of my gallbladder.

The tech had been called in for holiday and she was pissed. I could see her snarling as they brought me over for an asap Ultrasound. At first, she was looking and chatting. Then she got very kind and tender and asked me to roll over onto my belly.

I then knew she was looking at my liver from the backside. She gently asked me if I wanted a warm blanket and then she went to the phone and was talking in a muffled tone to someone. She said they wanted a stat CT of my abdomen and pelvis but she didn't tell me why. I knew something was up and probably terrible. I was alone and scared.

I was sitting in a chair when the doctor came in and said I had a huge adnexal tumor and some hepatic masses too.

I know adnexal means tumor filled ovary. I had done 2 journeys with nurses who had ovarian cancer etc. one of whom had died, one of whom is thriving. I immediately started bawling.. They asked me if I wanted my kids called.

My Daughter LaCie, who is a nurse, said she would be right there. My other daughter Gillian the policewoman arrived asap. My youngest Sparkie, said she would be right down and jumped in car from Maine. We were all blindsided.

They medicated me for pain, Anxiety, And nausea. It was quite the cocktail.

They sent me home to follow up with local cancer center.

We live 30 minutes from one of the top 10 cancer centers in the USA- Dana Farber. My daughter kept calling and calling until she got me a next day appt.

Because I was so short of breath, I went to my PCP to get some Xanax to help me deal. Normally I'm a fighter, but this was a tremendous hit. I got the script.

We all went to my first visit. The oncological surgeon said I was inoperable because the webbing was everywhere. According to the doctor, it was too dangerous to take these beasts out.

They were concerned that the cancer cells might seed into new sites.

My PCP wanted a good CT of the pelvis and abdomen with contrast, to check for spread   It showed over 15 masses in and around my liver, making surgery impossible. I had no symptoms of this slippery snake, ovarian cancer.

I got my port placed right before my second treatment. I was getting frontline therapy; taxol and carboplatin. 6 cycles, every 3 weeks. It's cumulative too. As the treatments go on, the symptoms can get worse.

I didn't care about losing my hair. It's only hair. But, all my body hair left too, and that was upsetting.

I had a great great team in Boston. The supportive care is the best part. They answer all texts and concerns very rapidly.

I did great with regard to support, but I was sick as a dog from the treatment.

For quite a while, I went from bed to shower to chair in my living room. I had 3 dogs. They stayed at my dude through it all. I was blessed. Then my little Westie started having seizures and I had to put him down one night around 4 am I was alone for that too. I howled like a wild wolf losing her cub.

My little corgi was having mobility issues so I had to carry her in and out whenever she needed to go out. As I got weaker and weaker that proved to be too much.

I'm Brca 2 positive. So my team used lynparza on me for maintenance meds post chemo, however I had lots of side effects with that nasty pill, including bone pain, massive fatigue, nausea, and aches and pains in all my joints. I found that medical marijuana was the best at combatting all those negative effects.

At the same time, I was going through upheaval in my living situation. I sold my home after 3 years of arguing with my ex. We split the monies and I moved to Maine to live with my daughter Hailey and her little family. It was great until my son in law and I started losing patience with each other. I was stubborn and obnoxious, I will admit.

 I found a very cute apartment about 40 minutes north of my daughter. About 1200 people live in the town; it's very quaint and artsy.

I moved in during a March blizzard, with help from my brother Ricky. It was so quaint with French doors into each bedroom. I was in love.

Initially, I felt great. I was taking all my meds as ordered, but then I started to change. I felt weird yet couldn't put my finger on it I made it through my first summer there and I loved it. The local food pantry kept me fed, and my brother's wife would always send good food home with me. My daughter LaCie paid my cable and Sparkie paid my cell phone bill. I had no other bills other than propane needs. I was glad summer was over because I can't tolerate the heat.

The insomnia was becoming quite severe by sept/October. I was intensely nauseous from the insomnia. I reached out to my Boston team. They ordered Compazine. It worked like a charm on the nausea, but another side effect was proving more difficult to control. I was peeing my pants. Another insidious symptom.

I spent a couple of days at my daughter's house playing with kids and though they said nothing they told me later that I was acting very strange. As it turns out, I had 2 seizures at her house. I said I think I'm having seizures and she kind of laughed like "symptom of the day mom"

I drove home around 2 pm and they kept asking me to stay because I was OFF. I opted to leave, but I had a very hard time staying in my right lane. I kept swerving over into the wrong lane. A lady behind me was beeping and flicking her lights at me. I got home and pissed my pants as I tried to get my keys in the door, so I jumped in the shower.

As i was finishing I felt my head shake and I watched my left arm shake and spasm. I said to myself I'm having a seizure. OMG. I need to get out of here safely. My dog was half in the shower so I reached down to grab her collar. She waited for me to safely step out of shower then she pulled me into living room.

I called my brother and he raced me to the local ER in a small hospital. They did the appropriate testing and ordered an MRI, which showed 2 large masses taking up my whole right hemisphere of my brain.

What a trip!!!!

So they sent me to Boston after determining just how serious this was. I was transported via a huge ambulance with three paramedics to Brigham and women's hospital for neurosurgeon consult and surgery. It was quite the ride. I remember it being very windy. I was very nervous. All my kids were called and met me at hospital.

My dog was brought to a sitters house and my 21 year old cat went to brother Ricky's house   My life was changing severely and I had no control over it. Again, this asshole cancer snuck into my life like a wrecking ball

I was refusing surgery because the tumor was causing cognitive issues. I was skipping appointments, lying to my kids, and I stopped taking my lynparza. I just didn't care. I even got into a car accident and lied thru my teeth about whole situation. This just wasn't me.

Post op: after neurosurgery was very tough. My days were filled with pain and confusion.

I was suicidal and admitted it, which allowed me to obtain help. I had an actual suicide plan. I was going to tie my weak leg to a cinder block and jump in the ocean. As I thought about it, I realized that drowning is a terrible way to go. Instead of harming myself, I set up counseling. I also made sure to have appropriate medications for when anxiety over-whelms me. Part of my healing was that I told my girls about all the lies I had told them.

After the grueling neurosurgery, I found that I can no longer drive. I walk with a cane, but I threw my walker to the side. I had my stitches out last week. It hurt like hell. We have a huge plan in place to kick this asshole cancer in the teeth again with Radiation the week of Christmas.(2023) Then one week off- then onto systemic chemo to smash all the little strays that think they may grow one day.

I'm living with my daughter, my 20 month old grandson, and my 3 month old Granddaughter.

I'm thankful to be alive. I no longer want to die. I Want to Live, Love and Laugh.

I'm pissed. I'm sad. But I'm not afraid.

I'm coming for you Cancer and I can't say it enough!!! I'm proud of myself because I survived. Now I have a plan for my continued life. All my ladies in support group are amazing and we lift each other up every minute.

I can't smoke marijuana again because the cough could injure my healing brain due to intracranial pressure. Like Gilda Radner stated- It's always something!

I do edibles, which work on my side effects without risking a stroke. My story ends with my battle. Radiation then chemo to kill this asshole cancer again; to steal more years. I was diagnosed Memorial Day 2019

My recurrence date was Nov 20th.

Surgery was the day before thanksgiving

My cancer loves holidays apparently.

Peace out. Lou

5

I AM THE STORM

BY MANDY RICHARDSON

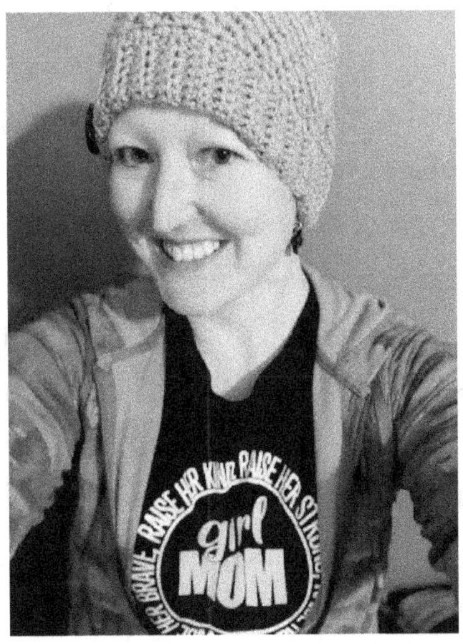

I t was May 2021. My daughters were 6 years old and 7 months old, and I was breastfeeding when I noticed the sore and pesky, but tiny, clogged duct. This wasn't my first baby, and this wasn't my first clog, so I decided to give it time. I massaged it. I used warm compresses. I nursed and pumped and pumped and nursed. But the knot got bigger. I started rethinking my self-diagnosis when I realized my flow hadn't been impacted at all, despite the increasing size of this clog, so in mid-June I made an appointment with my OB-GYN. The nurse practitioner felt it, as well as someone she was training, and they agreed it was a clogged duct. It felt "ductal" they said. It wasn't warm to touch, and I hadn't had a fever, so they suggested a few other techniques to help break it up and told me to give them a call if I got a fever.

I waited. All summer. There was never a fever. My flow was never interrupted. Sometimes I thought I felt like the knot was softer and that the massages were making progress. Warm water felt really soothing. But the lump was still getting bigger. I called back and asked to move up my annual appointment and was scheduled for the end of September. By then, the knot was visible under my skin and determined to be "angry" looking. I was 33. I was breastfeeding. And I didn't have a family history of breast cancer prior to menopause (I did have a pretty extensive one after, however). To top it off, the thing hurt. I was reassured when told cancerous tumors weren't usually painful. I was put on a pretty strong antibiotic for mastitis and told that it should clear up in 10 days.

I called back after 7 when there hadn't been any improvement.

I had been reasonably reassured up until that point, and while I was waiting to be seen again, I took my daughters to our local Autumn festival with several friends and their children. I remember describing the "knot" to my girlfriends as the size and shape of a lil' Smokies sausage. My baby turned one. We took a family trip to the Pennsylvania Grand Canyon. Hiking became painful, because my little one still rode in her pack-facing front.

I received a message from the oncology center shortly after we returned home from that trip. Livid, I put in a call to my NP before calling them back to schedule an appointment. Again, I was reassured that no one suspected cancer. The breast center was housed together with oncology, and they were the group next best suited to try to help me. I begrudgingly made my next appointment.

It was now late October.

I went into the office, where I was immediately reassured that it was an abscess and they could drain it then and there. I about cried in relief. By then, I felt like there was an increasingly heavy foreign object in my breast that was going to drop out at any moment. Two attempts to drain it with a rather large needle produced only blood return. When I was sent home with no relief, I did cry.

An ultrasound was finally ordered. It was confirmed that this supposed clogged-duct-turned-abscess was actually a solid mass. I was told over and over there still wasn't cause for concern. Lactating women developed benign masses reasonably commonly.

I was no longer reassured. But I didn't know enough to be scared at that point. The resident surgeon wanted to be the one to perform the biopsy, so another appointment was made, and back I went to the breast center 3 days later.

My breast cancer risk profile was incredibly low, I was reassured. Because it was now so large and close to the surface, the surgeon warned me that I would likely leak breast milk for some time while the biopsy site healed. I would hear from them sometime in the next week.

That weekend was Halloween. I took my girls camping with our family. We trick-or-treated through our neighborhood. I continued nursing my very stubborn almost 13 month old, who was still refusing bottles.

On November 2, 2021, my first grader had off school and was watching a movie in the living room. Her little sister, luckily, was napping, when I received the phone notification that my test results were available. I didn't hesitate to open it - although sometimes, in hindsight I wish I would have.

Invasive Ductal Carcinoma.

Grade 3.

There was a lot of other information. My mind could only focus on "carcinoma." I probably had a good half hour to google the rest before I received a call from the surgeon who had performed the biopsy. It was big. It was aggressive. They would probably want me to do chemotherapy first, but an oncologist would be calling me soon to set up an appointment. In the meantime, I scheduled an appointment for that Friday afternoon with the surgeon to touch base after I'd spoken with oncology.

The rest of that day passed in a blur. I couldn't react in front of the girls, especially my oldest. So I went out on to the front porch to call my husband, my mom, and a good friend who had gone through her own battle with breast cancer just the year before. I went back inside. I played with the girls and I finished my work day. I may have called my boss, I don't actually remember. I made a couple more calls to other friends that evening. My husband left work early and my parents made the hour drive up for dinner. There was no game plan. We didn't have much more information to go on, except that someone should be contacting me "soon."

We focused on something we could start to figure out: how to tell our 6 year old. How could we be honest but not scare the hell out of her? Especially when we were terrified ourselves.

I did a lot of reassuring over those next couple of days. I reassured my husband and my family that I would fight like hell. I would beat this. I would be the storm.

Was that true? I didn't know. How advanced was the cancer? How awful would treatment be? It didn't matter. I just knew I had to beat it.

But something else clicked. I was done waiting. Done waiting for someone to call me. Done waiting for someone else to figure out the answers for me. My mother in law was a nurse at Johns Hopkins, and happened to know a surgeon who could see me on short notice. I wasn't completely ready to commit to treatment in Baltimore rather than closer to home, so I called the breast center. I was informed that everyone was "just really busy" which was why I hadn't yet received a phone call from oncology, and I informed them I'd be by the next day to pick up my records. I canceled my Friday appointment, and instead my husband drove me to John's Hopkins to meet my new surgeon and medical oncologist.

The tumor was large, and very aggressive, as confirmed by my surgeon, Dr C. She had already requested the biopsy so that they could perform their own analysis of it. But she told me that morning that it was beatable. Because of its size, I would need chemo before she could operate. She had already spoken to the medical oncologist, whom I was on my way to meet next. As my husband and I sat in Dr. Cz office and she told me I would need to begin chemo before thanksgiving (2.5 weeks!) because we'd lost so much time, I realized we'd made the right decision to stop waiting. I didn't realize, at the time, how incredibly fast a timeframe that was, or that most people wait 5-6 weeks to a couple of months before beginning chemotherapy, and I asked if it would be OK to wait so long.

"A couple of weeks is OK", she told me, "A couple of months would not have been."

But I still needed testing. A lot of it. A PET scan, a mammogram, an ultrasound and an echocardiogram. In addition, I needed to be scheduled for my port placement. So I became the storm. I called, and I begged, and I called again and again to make sure I could get my appointments in before our target of the Wednesday before thanksgiving.

I was able to get my PET scan locally.

Then - another curveball. The PET scan detected activity around the lymph nodes in my armpit, which wasn't surprising. But it also picked up on something in the area of my right ovary. The activity was not as strong as my tumor, but it was stronger than in the lymph nodes. We completed bloodwork for breast cancer and ovarian cancer markers. As expected, the breast cancer marker came back high. Unexpectedly, so did the marker for ovarian cancer.

We didn't have time to think, not really. Dr Cz had gotten me an appointment with a gynecological oncologist for the day after she received the results. It was now November 17. It was surprisingly a relatively quick appointment. Was this ovarian cancer? Or was it a metastasis of the breast cancer? He didn't want to take the time to find out. It had to come out. His recommendation was to take my right ovary and both fallopian tubes, to limit any potential future occurrence or possible recurrence of ovarian cancer. He would biopsy after it was out. Getting me to chemo for the breast cancer was still the #1 goal. Understanding this, he scheduled my surgery for the next morning, November 18, and exactly one week before Thanksgiving.

My husband and I had a brief discussion of what this type of surgery meant: I would not be able to conceive any more children naturally. Ironically, our youngest was conceived through IVF in early 2020 after several miscarriages. We'd had 3 remaining embryos that we had decided to allow to be destroyed just that past summer. We didn't even consider the possibly of another egg harvest; this was sign enough for us that our family was complete. And how lucky we were to have our two beautiful girls before this all started.

I recovered in our basement, where it was quiet and I could put my feet up, and that location also gave me a little space from our baby, who I had to wean cold turkey in preparation for my upcoming treatment. During an afternoon nap, my husband came down and encouraged me to get up and move a little, suggesting I take my pain medicine and walk outside for a couple of minutes.

In front of our house were all of our neighbors, decked out in pink and holding signs of support. As I hugged and thanked them, a small fire truck drove up our hill, with my brother driving! Behind it were all of our families and friends, coworkers, and members of a car club that our neighbor belonged to. They were all decked out in pink balloons and paint, with their own flags and signs of support. It was incredible how the most nightmarish 2 weeks of my life could end on such a high note of love and support. My sister even packed up the girls and took them to her house for the night.

Dr F, the gynecological oncologist who performed my surgery, called the following Monday. There had been no mass that he could locate. The pathology from my ovary was benign. No one was sure what the PET had picked up on, but it wasn't cancer, and it wasn't going to get in the way of me starting chemo. While my medical oncologist wanted to give my body more time to recover, Dr F helped me advocate for beginning treatment the Wednesday before Thanksgiving. And that is exactly what I did.

I had my first adriamycin and cyclophosphamide (AC) treatment on November 23. Our neighborhood got together and arranged for everyone to bring us a different part of Thanksgiving dinner on Thursday. They covered everything, including dessert, because they were damned if they were going to let us order something, and we couldn't travel to our parents like we usually did.

They took it even further, though, and organized a meal train for Thursday-Sunday every week that I had treatment. Family members participated, and my coworkers filled in where someone hadn't been able to sign up. They brought goodies and other things to help comfort and relax, to help me take care of myself. They dropped off coloring books and puzzles that I could do while sitting in a chair for 3 hours during treatment. They brought toys and activities for my girls.

I was only briefly able to get out of bed on Christmas morning. My third AC treatment had been that Thursday. My hair had started falling out just before my second treatment, and a friend helped my shave it very short. I was taking my anti-nausea medication as prescribed, but I was completely zapped. My first hat was a soft festive hat with Santas all over it from my oldest daughter. I wore that to my third treatment and on Christmas morning. It took two full weeks to get all the presents wrapped and under the tree, but Santa came and we had breakfast together as a family before I had to return to bed.

I was gifted several more hats from friends, and I decided to try to wear a different hat to each treatment. It wasn't hard! Once people learned what I was doing, I was sent even more! It was just another incredible outpouring of support.

I had 4 total rounds of AC, followed by 12 weekly Taxol treatments. I finished in early April and had a few weeks to recover before surgery in May.

The weekend before my last treatment, my neighbor's car club held a fundraiser for our family. They invited us to their opening day, where I even got to pick the Mandy's choice recipient! They presented me with a check to help offset some of my medical costs, and to do something fun with the family!

We decided to take a family vacation to the Smoky Mountains in between treatment and surgery. We had to be careful; I was still immunocompromised. We cooked in, and ate at outdoor restaurants. But we could hike. My hair had started growing back a little, and my strength was slowly returning.

The original tumor had been 6cm. Post chemo testing showed that the disease had been shrunk to less than 1cm! We were able to scale back from me NEEDING a mastectomy to having a choice between the mastectomy and lumpectomy. Talk about a hard decision. I went back and forth multiple times, but because of the chemo response, my chances of recurrence in that breast were virtually the same. I talked to other women who had made that decision.

Having a toddler heavily weighed into my own decision. Had there been any kind of significant difference between the risk of recurrence, I would have chosen the mastectomy in a heartbeat. But when comparing the recoveries from each surgery, the mastectomy was much more daunting with a much longer lifting restriction, for an improvement of 1-2% in risk. I was also looking at needing radiation regardless of choice, because of my age. I spoke with women who opted for the mastectomy so they didn't have to go through radiation, but that wasn't my own game plan. I chose the lumpectomy and had my surgery on May 12, 2022.

"Give me one year" my surgeon had said at the start of everything. One year, and this would all be in the rear view mirror. So far it had been 6 months, and I was already moving in the direction of putting it all behind me. Dr C was able to confirm quickly that we'd gotten clear margins from surgery, but the pathology and staging took a couple of weeks.

I was staged at IIIa because of the size of my tumor. While my lymph node biopsy had come back negative, I'd definitely had at least one swollen lymph node that shrank after chemo, which lead to the speculation that there must have been some involvement. I had three removed at the time of my lumpectomy, and all 3 were negative for disease.

The residual disease pathology in my breast came back as Triple Negative. I started 30 rounds of radiation in July, wrapping up on my daughter's first week of second grade. I had a small break, then started an oral chemo called Xeloda, to further lower my risk of recurrence after learning of the TNBC diagnosis. I finished that in early February 2023 and started Tamoxifen in April.

The original biopsy of the breast tumor had come back with a slight Estrogen positive pathology. It was high enough, however, that my oncology team determined I could benefit from taking Tamoxifen.

I sometimes joke that I've gotten to experience a little bit of everything throughout my cancer journey.

As I write this, I have just passed two years since I finally received my diagnosis. Once I was able to wrap my head around what I was going through myself, I began advocating. Encouraging women to keep up on their annual exams. Knowing our own bodies. Don't take no and don't wait for an answer. Cancer doesn't discriminate. I've talked to women even younger than me with worse diagnoses. I joined a recently formed support group at Johns Hopkins to talk to other young women who had just learned of their diagnosis. I've connected to women through Facebook and other ways, sometimes just by being outspoken about my own diagnosis. Some people need their privacy, and that is to be respected. But I felt that I needed to scream my story from all the rooftops.

Hiking became my refuge. Being immunocompromised during the pandemic wasn't ideal, but we were careful. We kept our toddler out of daycare. My older daughter had to be cautious at school, but she developed a good group of friends who knew our situation and we were able to have carefully planned-out playdates. But I didn't have to worry about germs if I was hiking. I was even able to meet up with a friend from work to hike a couple of times. It was hard, as I was trying to not only get my energy back, but to get back in shape physically after treatment. Being outside made me feel better, both mentally and physically. Hiking continued to be something that our family could do together that allowed us to feel normal.

I don't know if I've actually helped anyone. But I know the way I felt when other women reached out to me. A stranger who knew someone who knew my aunt (who is also a survivor by the way!). A kind woman at the car show that I never got to speak with, but who passed me a shirt she'd made me with my new favorite quote:

"The devil whispered in my ear:

You're not strong enough to withstand the storm.

Today I whispered in the devil's ear:

I am the storm."

I had discovered that quote right after my diagnosis, and tried to live by it as I went through treatment. When I received the shirt, I knew it had meant something.

Another woman I met was my husband's coworker. I'm not sure exactly how it happened, but she had called him for something work related, and suddenly he was handing the phone off to me.

She and I talked and touched base with each other throughout our treatments, and then after. She was the one who learned of Camp Bravehearts, and invited me to try to join her for their weekend camp in August. I found out early on my diagnosis just how wonderful and strong the pink community was. But after attending my first Bravehearts camp, that was reinforced exponentially.

Every one of us has a story. And there's no need to compete with one another for "who had it worse." I've never felt that way among my pink sisters. Cancer sucks enough and we're all in each other's corners.

CANCER DOES NOT DEFINE ME

BY RUTH BURNS

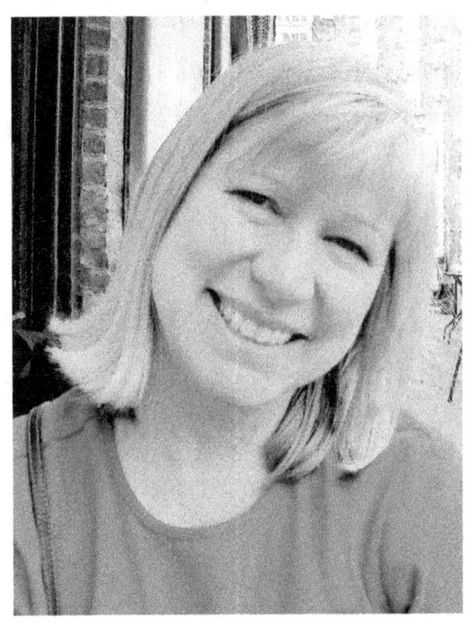

I t was 2008. My job as a billing and order clerk was ending. The company was going bankrupt after losing business to Asian companies. I had been there for 13 years. As a divorced mom with two kids, I needed to get a job ASAP. With the writing on the wall, I took the Civil Service test and interviewed for different positions. I took one at Children and Youth Services as a phone operator and just in time because my other job folded. Unfortunately, medical benefits wouldn't kick in for 3 months.

When I could finally use my benefits, I went for my mammogram. They saw something and sent me for an ultrasound. Again, the results were not good, so they sent me to have an MRI next. I needed a biopsy, but the insurance wasn't going to pay for it either. Stressed out and fighting with the insurance company, they finally said they would pay for the MRI. Then the doctor notified me that he wouldn't take any pay for the biopsy and would do it free of charge. He was super nice about it all. But soon I got a call from the MRI place while I was at work. I had CANCER!

So, the diagnosis was breast cancer in the left breast. Now I had a tough decision to make. Should I just remove one breast and take my chances the other side was fine? I really didn't want to have to go through the process again. I decided to have a bilateral mastectomy. For me, it seemed like the best option.

The surgery went well. Afterwards the worst part was the drains. They had to be emptied often and were uncomfortable. Luckily the drains were only in for about a week. I didn't want implants yet, so instead of doing that surgery, I wore these fake boobs filled with gel in my bras. They were no fun: sweaty and uncomfortable. Around this time, I also began getting hot flashes to add to the fun.

Next on the "Let's Beat Cancer" agenda was a visit to the oncologist. I was talked into doing chemotherapy. I made the decision but felt defeated about it. Although they did say they got everything from the surgery, they told me this was a precaution. I thought it would help me to get rid of any stray cancer cells. Chemo was hell. At least for me.

The first two treatments were not that bad but by the third and fourth I felt awful. I would have terrible migraines and my eyesight blurred. I could not be around any strong smells, and my nostrils burned. Especially bad were the odors from things like garlic, onions, cabbage, broccoli. I was crying and hoping to die. They took me off the chemo and said someone with a super strong sense of smell like me should have never done chemo. It was the worst experience of my life.

I also lost my hair, but that part wasn't so bad. I kinda liked it. It was easy to take care of and I hoped that maybe the chemo would change my hair when it re-grew. I had heard it sometimes did. I was born a blue-eyed blonde and never really liked it. Anyway, my hair came back blonde, but also curly! I always wanted curls! But they didn't last. It soon went straight again. There was nothing I liked about chemo...

The worst side effect of the chemo was hearing loss. It wasn't that bad at first, but it got worse. I now need to wear a hearing aid. It sucks. They said I'll have to learn to read lips. Good thing for closed captioning and texting. That really helps and my kids prefer it anyway.

I decided five years later to get breast implants and I can say I'm incredibly happy with the results. These won't wear out. I'll have the best boobs in the nursing home!

My cancer journey is still ongoing with the discovery of a recent melanoma on my leg. Thank goodness I don't need chemo. The best part, if there is any "best" part of my journey with cancer, is a group I joined called Camp Brave-hearts. I've made many new friends that are on their cancer journey, too. We go on trips, have adventures, talk and support one another. We have found strength in each other, comradery, and deep understanding. But mainly, we have the most fun just being together, celebrating each new day, and laughing. We have lots of laughs. Take that cancer!

I've decided that cancer does not define me but has enabled me to ask questions about my own health and to become proactive. I have true empathy for people with cancer and their caregivers. I also have accomplished many things since having cancer. I like traveling, (I love to snorkel, swim and kayak), I'm in a bowling league (and getting better, ha, ha), and I paint! I love to do watercolors! I've made a raised vegetable garden, I go to live musical concerts, and I see the latest movies. These are the things that define me, not cancer.

THE SUMMER OF 1990
BY ANDREA

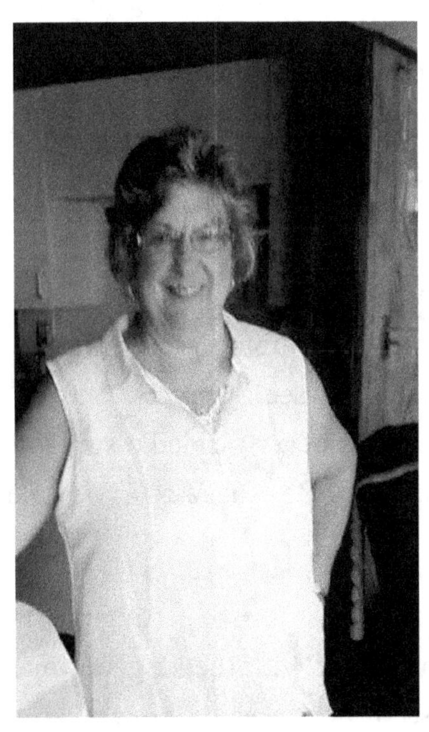

I t was the summer of 1990 and time for my yearly mammogram. A mammogram is not one of my favorite exams even though I know they are necessary. I was also diligent about giving myself self exams as well, which was a good thing because before I even got to the mammogram, something was different. I felt something new in my left breast.

I didn't think it was something (or was I hoping it wasn't?). I didn't say anything to anyone at first; I was just trying to talk myself into thinking that I was ok, after all I had 2 children to worry about. My daughter was only 8 years old. My son was 12 but boys react differently to girls with all this.

Of course, there is my husband who I knew would be there for me, but I had to tell him. Finally, I did, and his answer was "Did you call the doctor?" I said "No, not yet." His reply was "Well, you better!"

I called my family doctor and made an appointment we discussed options. A mammogram by itself wasn't an option, so he suggested that I see a surgeon and of course I didn't know who because I never needed a surgeon before. Fortunately, the surgeon he suggested was someone I had heard of.

All I could think was "So this is getting real now." My doctor made the appointment with the surgeon for me. When I got there, I could see how successful he was because the waiting room was filled with patients. Of course, as a new patient I had to fill out the paperwork and wait extra long to see him but in the end I knew he was the doctor who was going to do right by me. I had a biopsy done first before surgery to see if it was Breast Cancer and of course it was, and the lump that I thought was small was 4 centimeters, the size of a golf ball. The next step was surgery.

The surgery I had was a complete mastectomy of the left breast. My treatment afterwards was to take tamoxifen for 5 years which was suggested by my oncologist.

After I was healed, I needed to do something to give back. My daughter and I started to go to the local "Race for the Cure "every year. It was something we looked forward to doing together. By going to the yearly race, I met other women who also were cancer survivors. Up until then I had never known anyone affected by breast cancer. In 2003-2004, I found out through one of my daughter's friends there was a store that sold prosthetics, wigs, and garments called "That Special Woman" They are located in Ohio but have a website and ship all over the US. The store owner is related to my daughter's friend. I felt comfortable going there for these things. It was here I was introduced to the Bravehearts. I attended my first camp with Bravehearts in 2004 and have been going back as often as I can. Here I met countless women just like me. I was able to go and enjoy weekends away with these women and try out new experiences, like white water rafting, zip lining, and bonding. This gave me a much-needed sense of community and sisterhood.

STRONGER THAN THE STORM

BY ROBERTA DWYER

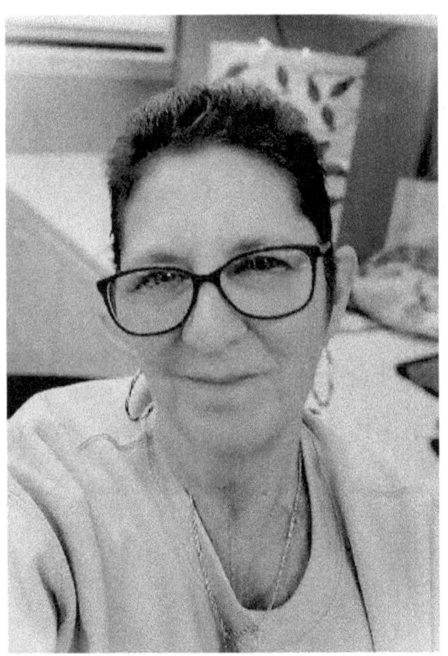

I wrote this chapter to leave a mark of my life for my children and granddaughter who are my strength and keep me fighting. I want to thank my mom, aunt, uncle, cousins, nieces, and friends for being my support, my cheerleaders and being there when I needed their care, love, and kindness.

This is a chapter of my journey for people who are, will or know someone who is going through the cancer journey. I hope this will open everyone's eyes that have not been through this journey or had a loved one that has been through this, to have compassion for the ones who are struggling through cancer.

THE BEGINNING

It was just the beginning of a new chapter of my life when I was diagnosed with breast cancer in my left breast on January 17, 2023, at the age of 54. Several years before, I was diagnosed with Ductal Papilloma which was noncancerous tumors that grew in my left breast milk duct. My surgeon at this time told me we caught this early before it turned into cancer. I had the tumors surgically removed and was told that there was nothing to be concerned about knowing they were benign and to continue my annual mammograms going forward.

In November 2022, I went for my annual mammogram. After my mammogram I received a call from the breast center stating my images showed some concern. I figured it was nothing, I have been going through health issues since I had Covid back 2020 which I had so many blood tests, MRIs and CTs on my body, what's another mammogram. If it was such a concern, why schedule me another mammogram in January 2023. Must not be that concerning.

January 4, 2023, I went to the breast center to get another mammogram. During my mammogram, I received multiple images and an ultrasound. I was asked to get dressed and sit in the waiting room; the doctor's assistant will come in to discuss what's next. I sat there with overload of emotions, fear of the unknown. The doctor's assistant came into the room and told me they needed to do a biopsy on two masses and scheduled it for the following week. I walked out of the hospital shaking and crying. Fear of going through another biopsy knowing I wasn't the best patient last time, I fainted during that one so now my fear has taken over before this procedure is performed. I was more worried about the biopsy than the outcome of the results because I felt the tumors would be benign and they would just put markers in to monitor, during my annual mammograms going forward.

January 9, 2023, I went for my biopsy. I had my daughter bring me to my appointment knowing I needed to take Xanax that was prescribed to me for the procedure so my anxiety wouldn't get the best of me. Xanax didn't help and again I fainted after the first biopsy.

All was a success of the biopsy, and they sent me home. Now, it was the waiting game for the results. While waiting for results, I continued to check the patient portal and the mail to just have something saying biopsies were benign. No news is good news, right?

Eight days later, on January 17, 2023, while at work, I received a call from the doctor telling me she had good news and bad news. One tumor was benign, but the other tumor was cancer. The doctor said she will refer me to a surgeon, and I would be contacted ASAP. I was so overwhelmed with emotions, sitting in a conference room at work. I called my mom crying hysterically, not knowing how I was going to deal with this. What's going to happen to me? Will I be able to handle this? How bad is the cancer in my breast? What is the stage of cancer? How will I tell my adult children? How will this affect my granddaughter, her MiMi being sick? My heart was breaking with this news.

I'm a single 54-year-old woman and don't have a spouse to support me through this. My daughter and granddaughter live with me, and I don't want them to be burdened with this. I don't want them to see me sick and go through this terrible disease.

I have been a strong woman all these years, a military wife, divorce, single mom of two children, worked 2-3 jobs to support myself and children to make ends meet. Now I don't have control of my life. I can't just push this to the side and keep moving as I have done throughout my life.

BREAKING THE NEWS TO FAMILY

After leaving work early that day, not remembering the drive home, knowing my thoughts were consumed of the news of having cancer.

How do I tell my adult children I have breast cancer. They have seen what cancer does, between me losing a dear friend who was diagnosed with breast cancer at the age of 40 and passed away at the age of 48 after being in remission for 5 years and 3 uncles who passed away from prostate cancer. I was so worried about them, more than myself, about how they would handle the news. They saw me as a strong mother, the rock of the family.

I called my son and told him my diagnosis. I honestly can't remember our phone conversation; I know he was upset, concerned, and had many questions that I couldn't answer. Now, I had to wait until my daughter got home from work. When she walked through the door, she looked at me and asked me what's wrong. I told her I got my results back and I have breast cancer. She broke down immediately and I embraced her letting her know I would be OK. I'm not going anywhere, and I will fight this.

Honestly, deep down inside, will I be able to fight this and how long will I have in life going forward knowing of the unknown. But I had to be the strong mother my children have seen their whole life.

After telling my mom and children, it was time to tell my close family members and friends. All I remember is repeating the same story to each of them. I was exhausted and completely shut down.

From that day, I created a private Facebook group for my family and friends. Instead of having 15-20 people contacting me daily, I posted and shared information and updates on my journey through breast cancer. It can get overwhelming receiving texts and repeating updates to everyone through different text chains. I also forgot at times to keep everyone updated on things because of the over-whelming emotions involved which made me feel guilty. Yes, it might seem strange that I felt guilty, but I always think of everyone else before myself.

I know I am loved and have a great support system. I now need to focus on what's next.

Suggestion: This is something to consider doing if you are on social media. I was able to post about my appointments, treatments, emotions, my treatment side effects, etc. Doing this I received so much support from my close friends and family. It kept my spirits up and continued to fight.

My Diagnosis

My primary doctor called me later that afternoon and told me I was diagnosed with Triple Negative Invasive Ductal Carcinoma grade 2-3. She referred me to a doctor within the healthcare group she is associated with so she would be able to be part of my cancer journey and help me when needed. After I hung up with my primary doctor and started researching the diagnosis. I kind of got an understanding of what type of cancer it was but looking at survival rate, etc. made things worse for me.

So, what is Triple Negative Invasive Ductal Carcinoma grade 2-3? Invasive Ductal Carcinoma (IDC) is an invasive cancer where abnormal cancer cells that began forming in the milk ducts have spread beyond the ducts into other parts of the breast tissue. Triple Negative is negative for estrogen, progesterone and HER2. The grade of cancer is how fast the cancer is growing. Triple-negative breast cancer (TNBC) accounts for about 10% to 20% of all breast cancer cases.

I'm thinking to myself, great, of course I would get the worst type of breast cancer, why couldn't it be hormonal. Yes, I reminded myself that it was caught early, and the tumor was at this time at 1.6 cm.

Suggestion: Don't use Google doctor. I was told multiple times from the doctors and nurses. I have learned that the more you Google diagnoses and treatments the more you get scared, and I felt like this is a death sentence. When I did my research, I wrote down questions to ask the doctors. Make sure you write down your questions because when you meet with the doctors you will forget things.

CONSULTANTS AND TESTS

The night of the day I got the news, I received a call from a doctor of the breast center I got the mammogram and biopsy from. The doctor called me while he was home with his children in the background asking me to schedule an appointment with him the next morning. This seemed very strange to me. Why call me in the evening and from home with that distraction. At this time, I was still numb with the news and knowing my primary doctor already suggested one of the top breast surgeons in the capital area in my healthcare group, I tried to decline but he was determined. I agreed to meet with him the following morning just to get off the phone. I then was thinking to myself, this doctor seemed like an ambulance chaser. I looked up his medical information and he was just a general surgeon, and I couldn't find any information about him working with breast cancer patients. I called the next morning and canceled the appointment.

I received a call the following morning from a referred surgeon who is a highly recommended doctor that only works with breast cancer patients to set an appointment. They couldn't get me in ASAP knowing she was on vacation. I had a girl's trip planned for my 55th birthday to Florida the following week. They wanted to schedule me that week I was gone. I was going to cancel my trip, but my primary doctor told me not to cancel my trip. I should go on my trip to get away because the next 6 months will be a hard journey and I need to take this time to enjoy life. I took her advice.

The ocean air, sound of the ocean waves, the sunshine and sunrise were so needed and glad I went because February was the month everything started.

The first appointment was with my surgeon on February 2nd. I had one of my good friends go with me knowing I was told to have someone go to each appointment with me to take notes. I'm so glad I did take that advice because again, it was a blur. I thought the surgeon was going to just tell me that I needed surgery and that would be it. Nope, that wasn't the case. I will need lumpectomy, chemotherapy, and radiation. I needed multiple tests, MRI, CT scans and nuclear body scans to make sure it hadn't spread to any other parts of my body and to size the tumor to make sure it didn't grow bigger. This would determine what would come first, chemotherapy or lumpectomy. I was also referred to genetic counseling and testing due to my tumor characteristics and family history of cancer. The genetic testing would test for BRCA1 and BRCA2 gene.

My head was spinning walking out of the consultation. I'm thinking to myself, this is serious. All I kept seeing was my friend going through chemotherapy, seeing movies and commercials about cancer. I was scared to death. I kept thinking, why is this happening to me. What did I do wrong. I was anger as hell. I have the biggest heart, always helping people when needed, thinking of people before myself and accepting people for who they are with flaws and everything. I felt like I was being punished.

Suggestion: Always have someone go with you to every appointment. Have them take notes and ask questions they have that you missed or didn't think of asking. As a patient, we tend to focus on the bad news instead of all the other information that is provided. The information you receive at each appointment is very overwhelming.

February 8th, I had my pre-op appointment and oncologist consultation. My pre-op went well and was signed off for surgery. The oncologist consultation didn't go well. The oncologist was an hour late, which made me upset. I had to check in 20 minutes early for my appointment and then have me wait an additional hour. Once I got to see the doctor, she handed me the two chemotherapy medications information packages and told me not to read they may cause death. I thought to myself, "what the hell, is this a joke" and continued to say I will lose my hair and she will give me a script. She seemed unconcerned and going on with business. This isn't normal for me. I don't know what to expect but this doctor isn't for me. I had so many questions. I wanted to know more about this type of cancer, what chemotherapy will do to me and what are the side effects and long-term side effects, etc. I left the appointment and immediately called my primary doctor asking her if there was another doctor I could get referred to because if I have an oncologist for the next 15 years of my life, I want someone I feel comfortable with not someone that just made me feel like a number. My primary referred me to another oncologist within the group.

February 9th, I had the nuclear body scan, everything looked good, cancer didn't spread.

February 14th, I had a breast MRI and chest CT scans. Results of CT scan looked good no issues, breast MRI confirmed the tumor didn't grow and is still at 1.6 cm, less than 2cm which considered me a good candidate for lumpectomy first. Thank God, this was good news especially having TNBC.

February 15th, I had my radiologist consultation. He is an amazing doctor, very detailed and explained so much to me even outside of his area. He was able to look at my nuclear body, CT and MRI scans and explained everything to me. He gave me so much more information about my cancer, surgery, and treatments. He put me at ease with everything he said. I felt blessed to have him on my team. The next time I would see him would be 4 weeks after my last chemotherapy treatment which would be in July. I need 19 radiation treatments. Normally, they do 15 treatments but knowing I have TNBC, an additional 4 treatments will be added to target where the tumor was. Before I left my appointment, I voiced my concern about the oncologist that was assigned to me, and he told me he and my primary doctor will get a different oncologist. He understood my concerns and agreed I need to have someone I feel comfortable with. At this appointment I also found out that the surgeon, oncologist, and he meet every Thursday morning as a group to discuss patients. This was a big relief. I'm putting my life in their hands.

February 21st, I had counseling with Ferre Genetics. We went through my diagnosis and family history of cancer. I also provided them with one of my family members' genetic testing documentations for their review. I agreed for them to not only just test for BRAC1 and BRAC2 genes but to test for other mutant genes. I wanted to make sure that there wasn't anything else I needed to be concerned about and if something did come back positive my children and brother could get a genetic tested. I received a genetic kit via FedEx. I had to provide saliva in a tube and send it back to them via FedEx. Received my results back on March 13th and the results were negative. My cancer is environmental.

Suggestion: Always advocate for yourself. Don't just accept what is giving to you. If you don't feel the doctor is right for you, you don't connect, continue to push for what you want.

Surgery

I was scheduled for tracer injection of radiation on February 22nd and surgery on February 23rd. Before my scheduled procedures, I had to get the COVID test. Two days later the test came back positive. I was so upset, now surgery was pushed out 3 more weeks and I must isolate myself. Not sure where I got COVID. I have been working in the office 50% and been very careful around people.

My job offers reasonable accommodation to work 100% telecommuting. This program is required by the NYS Human Rights Law and the Americans with Disabilities Act (ADA). I wanted to apply for this, so I didn't get sick again for the next surgery date. I didn't want to push the surgery out again because of the cancer being aggressive and growing more. My fear took over because I'm ready for the treatment that has been selected for me and don't want to have it changed or the cancer to spread. I thought, will it spread that quick, I had no idea, but I wasn't going to chance it. I had to go through so much paperwork and communication with the office that handled these requests. My surgeon submitted everything they requested, and I kept getting communication from the office asking for more information. I felt they didn't care what I was going through and that my cancer is just a normal thing. I finally was approved weeks later. This process stressed me out so much and I cried multiple times at the frustration it caused.

With the downtime I had before my next scheduled surgery in March, I was advised to get my legal matters in order. I never thought about that. This hit me hard. I did a health proxy, power of attorney, and emergency power of attorney for my retirement. During this downtime, I found a book called 'Dear Cancer, Beating Triple Negative Breast Cancer' by Ann Tracy Marr. I felt like I was reading my journey when reading her words. The information in the book was very helpful and started getting some insight of TNBC. At that time, I had so many emotions; fear, anger, depression, being isolated and alone, I couldn't understand why she wrote Dear Cancer, I would of wrote F@ck Cancer. There is nothing dear about cancer. Three weeks as passed, it's time for surgery.

March 13th, I had radiation injection for nodes and TRAC in my left breast for tumor removal. My procedure consisted of injecting 2 needles of radiation in the nipple, in two different areas without any numbing. After that, they did a mammogram of it to make sure everything looked correct. Once verifying it was correct, they added another piece to the mammograph machine that pinpointed the area where the doctor needed to insert TRAC. Knowing I had 3 markers in my breast from biopsies, they had to pinpoint the correct one. After they found the correct marker, they injected numbing medication with needle, once numbed they put line in to place transmitter TRAC in for surgery. I'm not sure if I'm the only one that thinks this, but why is this procedure so uncomfortable. Again, my anxiety and pain from this, I almost fainted again. I was sent home and glad that part was over.

March 14th, surgery was performed at 10:55am. The surgery went well. During the recovery, I was in a lot of pain which I had to receive a high dose of morphine which caused nauseous, and I had to stay a little longer in recovery room than expected. I was released and got home around 4:00pm.

The next couple days were a little rough sleeping due to the pain and not being able to sleep on my left side. I experienced nerve pain from the lymph nodes excision which was commuted to me that this would happen. I didn't have a recliner and was sleeping in a normal bed. I had read in the book, Dear Cancer, that if you are going through this journey, you should invest in a recliner. A good friend of mine ordered and coordinated the delivery of a recliner a week after surgery. I wished I had this before surgery, but it did come in handy for the next 4 months.

Received results of surgery, lymph nodes biopsy was negative, tumor and breast tissue margins are clear. Thank God, no more surgeries and the cancer didn't spread. This was awesome news. If the breast tissue margins weren't clear, I would have had to get another surgery.

Now to the next step of this journey, chemotherapy.

Suggestion: If you don't have a recliner or something like one. You should invest in one. This will make your life a lot more comfortable.

TREATMENTS

As I said previously, I wasn't happy with the oncologist that was assigned to me. During my recovery time from surgery, I reached out to my primary doctor and radiologist following up on a new referral. The doctor they referred me to accepted me as a patient.

March 22nd, I had my appointment with the new oncologist. She was very thorough and very informative. She explained everything and answered all my questions. I started chemotherapy on April 12th. I received Taxotere and Procytox. I was told these drugs were very strong and have a lot of side effects. I had to get 4 treatments that were scheduled every 3rd week. I was given steroids before and after the day of chemotherapy, nausea medication and Neulasta Onpro to help with my white blood count. The oncologist put in a request to have the tumor tested for PD-L1 protein and to see what the percentage it was, to see if I would be a good candidate for immunotherapy treatment after chemotherapy.

What is PD-L1? The way it was explained to me was, this protein blocks T-cell activation to fight cancer cells. If my protein is higher than 60% I would be a good candidate for immunotherapy treatment and the doctor would have to request approval from my insurance company knowing treatment is very costly. My results came back with an 80%. Again, great, my immune system sucks and this news sets me back to when I heard I had cancer. But I will continue to stay positive and get my mindset ready for my first chemotherapy treatment.

During my visit with the oncologist, I asked about port placement. When I did my research on chemotherapy, it was suggested to get a port rather than a vein, eliminating the need for needles sticks and get a port placed in during chemotherapy. The oncologist agreed and scheduled me for the procedure before chemotherapy.

April 5th, I had the port surgically placed in my chest. My emotions got the best of me. While the nurse was prepping me, reality hit me hard. I broke down crying. I was scared and nervous of the unknown. Once they brought me in the surgical room, tears continued to flow. The nurses were very understanding and tried to comfort me. That night was rough. I wasn't prepared for this pain. I didn't think it was going to be that bad, but I was wrong. It was so uncomfortable after the numbing block wore off. I was prescribed pain meds, but I couldn't get relief. I was so happy that my friends purchased a recliner for me to sleep in because I needed to sleep straight to keep my neck in a straight position and place pillows under my arms, so I didn't accidently roll on the side the port was placed in. I was having neck pain and pulling feeling from the port and tube going up my neck which felt uncomfortable and was scared that I did something wrong, so I called the doctor and was told this is a normal feeling. During this time of healing, I kept thinking to myself, if I'm uncomfortable and freaking out with this, how the hell am I going to deal with my first chemo treatment. After a couple of days, I started feeling better. I was able to enjoy Easter with my children and granddaughter before my first chemotherapy treatment.

Suggestion: Things to have on hand before chemotherapy; baby wipes, Desitin, MiraLAX, Imodium A-D, Tylenol, ibuprofen, crackers, protein shakes, biotin mouthwash.

April 12th, I received my first chemotherapy treatment. Before going to the hospital, I had to apply Lidocaine on the port 30 minutes before the nurse accessed the port. I saw the oncologist before I received treatment to go over treatment again and to go over any questions I had. The nurse drew blood to make sure blood levels are good to go forward with the treatment. After 45-minute wait, I was cleared to start treatment. The nurse started saline drip and steroids before I received my treatment of docetaxel (Taxotere) and Cycolphosphamide (Cytoxan). For the first time of chemotherapy treatment, they had to start with a small dose going through IV to make sure I wouldn't get an allergic reaction for each drug. After treatment was over, the nurse placed Pegfilgrastim (Neulasta Onpro) device on my arm. This whole process was 5 hours long and very draining emotionally of the unknowns. I had a good friend go with me which made the time pass by quickly. We left the hospital and I felt good which I thought to myself this is good, maybe I won't have too many side effects. I was happy it was over told myself 1 down and 3 more to go. My friend stayed with me overnight just in case I needed help. I didn't sleep very well knowing the steroids had kept me up.

April 13th, I woke up with body aches, headache, and nausea. I started taking the instructed medications from the doctor.

Dexamethasone (Decardron) 1 tablet 2 times a day after treatment for one day, Ondamsetrom (Zofran) 1 tablet every 8 hours post chemo for 7 doses for nausea and Procholoperazine (Compazine) 1 tablet every 6 hours if needed for nausea. The Pegfilgrastim device went off later that day. This is used to treat neutropenia (low white blood cells) that is caused by cancer medicines. It reduces the chance of infection by receiving chemotherapy medications that may decrease the number of neutrophils. The device has a blinking green light, a beeping sound goes off and the medicine starts to inject in the body. The injection lasts 45-60 minutes. When it is completed, a long beep sound goes off and the light turns solid green, this is when you can remove it from your arm. This made me a little nervous not knowing what to expect, so I waited for my daughter to come home from work to remove it. I still had energy and used it to my advantage to do things while I can.

The next day was hell. I had multiple effects, migraine, constipation, nausea, body aches, facial flushing, and loss of appetite. It felt like I had the flu but times 10 worse. Constipation was so bad that I was on the floor in the bathroom crying and couldn't move. It felt like I was having labor pain. I have never experienced constipation like that in my life. My cousin had called me and drove to my house and brought MiraLAX knowing I didn't have any on hand and I couldn't drive to get any. After an hour of taking MiraLAX, my stomach was feeling so much better but still had other side effects. I was able to deal with the side effects other than the migraine. I couldn't get any relief with medications. On the following day, it was worse, I started to get nervous, worried about blood clot in brain, etc. I called the on-call doctor and suggested I go to the ER. I was brought to the ER, got blood work, CT scan of brain and X-ray of chest, everything was clear. The doctor side this might be a side effect of the chemo drug that is triggering my migraines and suggested that I talk to my oncologist at the follow up appointment that is scheduled in 4 days.

April 17th, my headache was subsiding, body aches and pain were manageable. I tried to eat food, but the food started tasting different and was losing my appetite. I started to get mouth sores, so I contacted the nurse coordinator, and she told me to make mouthwash of salt, baking soda and water and get biotin mouthwash for dryness. These remedies helped. I started to get very discouraged and wanted to quit. I didn't feel like I could continue to go through more treatments. This was only the beginning of this treatment and I had read that every treatment gets worse. I cried every night, prayed to my dad, who is no longer with me, to help me get through this and give me the strength I need to fight. Being single and not having someone to hold me during this time was a very lonely time of my life. I cried at night just wishing I had someone to hold me and say everything would be okay.

April 19th, I seen my oncologist for a follow-up. We discussed my side effects and drew blood to monitor my blood levels from previous blood work the week before.

Blood work was as good and no issues. My oncologist cleared me for my next treatment on May 3rd. My oncologist was shocked that I hadn't started losing my hair yet. I was hoping it wouldn't, maybe I would be the lucky one. But of course, I wasn't, the following week, and started to lose my hair. A few hairs here and there but then a couple of days later, brushes full of hair. My scalp and hair follicles were so sensitive. I guess it was time to shave my head. I reached out to my hairdresser and scheduled an appointment for him and have a group of my family and friends come and support me. The day of the appointment, I received a call from my hairdresser, he had covid. So, my cousin had clippers and my niece took the lead of cutting and shaving my head. My friends and family came over to my house and the ones who couldn't join in person Facetime to be by my side and help me cope. Tears were shed but laughter also lightened the moment. This was a very emotional time for everyone but noticed it hit hard for my daughter. I see tears flowing down her face while she was holding the phone facetiming for family/friends not present. It broke my heart to see her cry because she is like me, we don't cry in front of people, we hide our emotions.

May 3rd, I had my second treatment. My son brought me to the appointment. The doctor and I went over all my side effects, and she decided to decrease docetaxel (Taxotere) dosage knowing it was causing neuropathy and my body can't handle the high dose. I started dropping things and losing balance when walking. I honestly thought it was because of the treatment and being weak and tired. I didn't think it was neuropathy. I was told about neuropathy before getting treatment but totally disregarded it or was it the brain fog, I was experiencing.

During my treatment I was told to eat ice chips when receiving the chemotherapy drugs to help with mouth sores and taste which helped. This treatment started making me tired, weak, achy, visual migraine and uncomfortable not like the last time, I felt fine during treatment. I went home, again I had a friend stay with me overnight to make sure I was okay during the night. During the next couple days, I couldn't sleep, started getting a headache again but this time I started taking Ibuprofen to take the edge off which helped, neuropathy got worse, dropping things, legs seem to give out at times and was losing my breath when walking up and down the stairs and not being able to continue my bladder. I noticed brain fog started to kick in more, started to boil water on gas stove to cook some noodles and totally forgot about it. An hour later I noticed I did that, and the water evaporated. I decided not to cook when alone.

This time, my granddaughter wouldn't leave my side. I was sleeping in the living room on the recliner, and she slept on the couch. She was my little helper through this. She would bring me water, make me peanut butter, jelly sandwiches and bring me snacks. She was my strength, the reason why I was fighting. At the age of 5, seeing her MiMi sick, broke my heart. She has lived with me since she was born and we are very close, as a second mommy as my grandmother was to me when I was growing up. I never wanted her to see this or ever experience this in her life. At one point, she started crying and told me she feared me. She was scared that she would hurt me if she touched me. What a heartbreaking moment. She had asked me what I did wrong to get cancer and why do I have cancer. I had to explain to her in a way she could understand.

Suggestion: If you have children or grandchildren, there are books about someone you love who has cancer for children. I brought the book 'What happens when someone I love has Cancer? Explain the science of cancer and how a loved one's diagnosis and treatment affects a kid's day to day life.

During this 2nd round of treatment, it was challenging but more emotional. I had no energy and when I pushed myself to do things, such as normal things around the house, little gardening, walking around the neighborhood I got so exhausted and the next day I couldn't do anything because I was achy and had chills. It was so frustrating and made me depressed. I kept reminding myself bad days are followed by good days. I needed to pound it in my brain when I felt defeated.

I tried to do normal things like go to the store for a couple items, get gas, go through drive thru for food, etc. and people look at me with pity or what is her story. I didn't know what they were thinking, but it made me feel uncomfortable because I was wearing a bandana and only one wearing a mask which brings more attention to me. I wanted to tell them to stop staring. During this time, I put my retirement papers, I turned 55 in January and worked 31 years for the State Government. My job was the only normal thing in my life right now, but I was taking a lot of time off which goes towards your final retirement income and reduces my health insurance. I wanted to focus on my health plus not knowing what to expect after treatment. This was a big decision in my life, I didn't know if I could live on the retirement check monthly, but I pushed myself to retire, and my last day was May 31st.

May 24th, round 3 of treatment, my mom flew in from Florida to go with me and stay for a week to help me out. This treatment kicked my ass. I started feeling side effects a couple hours after treatment. I woke up in the middle of the night sweating, nauseous, bladder and stomach issues. I thought to myself, I normally don't feel like this so quickly. What the hell is the weekend going to feel like. The 2-3 days after treatment was hell. I talked to my oncologist about being fatigued all the time and how long I was down for the 2nd round. I was told this is expected and this treatment probably will be longer. This treatment was hell, my bones ached so much even just texting people hurt. I felt like death took over my body. I had issues eating and my go to food during chemotherapy makes me nauseous. I wanted to eat to get my energy back and feel better. I wanted to cry but didn't have the energy to do that. I laid at night in a fetus position to take away the discomfort. I had no one to talk to or hold me, I was so alone and scared. After 6 days, I started feeling normal again. I was still tired and had stomach issues, but I have gotten used to that and was manageable. I will take over the hell I experience.

May 31st, I noticed something poking out of my skin near the port placement. I contacted the doctor and had to go to the hospital for the doctor to look at it and to determine if it was a stitch or piece of the chest port. It was the knot of the stitch that didn't dissolve, and my skin rejected. Simple little procedure, and stitch was removed.

June 4th, round 4 my last chemotherapy treatment. I was feeling a little off, tired, and almost fainted while nurse inserted the IV tube in my port to get bloodwork done. Bloodwork numbers were fine and signed off to complete this treatment. During my appointment, my oncologist stated she will submit my paperwork to my insurance company for immunotherapy treatment (Keytruda). She stated that immunotherapy treatment will push out cancer relapsing. It troubled me hearing the word relapse. It was the first-time hearing this. I know there is a chance of the cancer coming back but I guess I was wishing not to hear the work relapse. After my treatment was completed, I got to ring the bell when I left with the nurses all clapping 'There is always something to be thankful for'. Again, this treatment was rough and with more of a punch. I fell asleep for a couple hours that night and woke up with side effects like the 3rd treatment but worse. It took me down for 5 days and had a couple more new side effects, switching in eyes, aura migraines and a little heart racing. I thought positively and told myself you are strong and get through this. This is the last time feeling like this, no more chemotherapy.

RADIATION TREATMENT

June 21st, I had radiation oncology follow-up appointment. Doctor and I went through everything we discussed back in March. I had to get a CT scan and tattoo markings before radiation treatment started. I was told knowing my cancer is in the left breast, the radiation could hit the heart, lung, and ribs, but with the newest technology, it decreased the chances of damaging the organs. The ribs will be damaged either way making left side more fragile and will need to be careful if I fall, etc. There were other health issues that my doctor went through to, but I wasn't very concerned about. My body is already taxed from chemotherapy. What else could happen. This would be a breeze.

June 28th, I had my appointment with the radiation oncologist to get my tattoo markings to start radiation treatment in 2 weeks. I got 6 tattoo markers which I thought was only going to be 4. The placing of the tattoo markings didn't hurt, but I did previously had gotten professional tattoos, so I knew what to expect. The radiation test run was scheduled for July 10th to verify the markers are in the right place.

July 11[th,] I had my first radiation treatment. It was a bit scary of the unknown but once I had the first treatment, the rest were fine. Radiation treatment was Monday-Friday, 20 minutes per visit, 5 minutes per treatment for 19 treatments. I was told to wash with non-sensitive dove soap, do not put deodorant on, and use Aquaphor to keep the skin moist and wear tank tops, no bras because it would irate the skin and might cause issues.

Before going into the radiation room, I had to undress waist up and put a gown on. I had to disrobe in front of my technicians which was a little uncomfortable, but I had concluded that my breasts are only anatomy and not to feel embarrassed. I had to lay down on my stomach and place my left breast in a hole and get positioned for the radiation treatment. Each day I went, it got easier. The technicians would put on music while I was in the room alone for treatment. I would sing in my head and count the number of songs for the treatment to be done. After the first week, I had the sound of the radiation machine down to the sounds to be completed. At one of my treatments, I told the technicians I was going to a Van Halen cover band that night, when they closed the door to start my treatment, they played Van Halen song Jump. I thought to myself, this team is amazing. They really do listen.

I can't express enough that the team was amazing, I'm always greeted by all the staff and socialize, it's like walking into work and talking about your day and what your plans are for the weekend. I was treated like I was part of their team. They were the most attentive, supportive, and thoughtful team. They made my experience easy. I also met other cancer patients that were going through radiation and talked about their journeys. Some were encouraging, but some were very sad.

The 10th radiation treatment, the doctor did scans to verify everything was looking good and confirmed radiation was working as expected. During this visit, I broke down crying in the waiting room. The nurses pulled me into a patient room and talked to me. The nurse referred me to the social worker. I was an emotional mess, anger and depression kicked in. During the past 7 months, I have been stuck in the house and not be able to live my life. I retired early, not traveling, being isolated, being sick, having no energy, being in pain and seeing other cancer patients struggling. During this whole time, I didn't cry or show any emotions knowing I was taught to be strong and keep moving. Well, this day, I couldn't shake it off like I have all these months.

I received a call from the social worker, and I agreed to start treatment. The social worker reached out to Aptihealth to get me scheduled with a psychologist. I was a little weary of this but maybe this will help me navigate through my anger and fear of cancer. It took over 6 weeks to find the right therapist but I'm now glad I did. I meet with my therapist every 2 weeks and I'm still currently having sessions. My therapist induced me to a group called Camp Bravehearts

Oncology Camp for Women. I joined the group. I'm still new to the group and hope to meet women when I attend the camps who have gone or going through the same journey I'm going through.

During my 19 treatments, I experienced energy level declining after the 2-weeks, irritation of skin which steroid cream was prescribed, and tenderness and nerve pain where the incisions were all normal side effects.

August 4th, my last radiation treatment. I received my certificate of completion. I can now say I'm in remission. It's time to heal physically, emotionally and continue my immunotherapy treatments.

IMMUNOTHERAPY TREATMENT

July 11th, I had my first immunotherapy treatment the same day of my first radiation treatment. I met with the oncologist to discuss the treatment, Keytruda, and had to do bloodwork to check blood count before getting treatment. The treatment only takes 30 minutes which is a blessing knowing chemotherapy took 3+ hours. I will receive treatment for the year, treatment is every 3 weeks.

August 1st, I had my second immunotherapy treatment. I had plans to travel to California during the next treatment, so my oncologist increased my dose to do it every 6 weeks instead of every 3 weeks. I traveled to California for a week with a friend to visit my family, to feel alive and some normality. It was a nice break from treatments and from my environment. Now, it was the best thing for me physically, probably not, but mentally it helped me feel some normality and was able to see my family which made me happy.

September 12th, I had my third immunotherapy treatment. I went by myself for the first time through this whole journey, I was in a funk, dealing with fatigue and not wanting to be around people. On this day, I found out my oncologist is leaving and going to work with a team on cancer research. I was sad because she is a great doctor and felt confident with my life in her hands, especially knowing I will have to have an oncologist for the next 15 years. She agreed to continue to see me through my immunotherapy treatments until July 2024. I will need to get assigned to a new doctor after treatment. The doctor and I agreed to do treatments every 6 weeks instead of every 3 weeks to help me mentally. When going to the cancer center, it gets very emotionally draining and the continue reminder of my cancer journey.

LIVING NOW

I'm now into the 10th month of this journey, my life is still overtaken by breast cancer, emotionally and physically. When looking in the mirror, I have the reminder of cancer, the loss of my hair and still have the chest port in. My hair is growing, I have maybe a little of an inch but at least I'm not bald anymore. Chest port for my immunotherapy treatments that won't be removed until after my last treatment in July

2024 which I need to remind myself that getting this treatment may push out cancer relapsing. I'm still experiencing fatigue, neuropathy and have been diagnosed with lymphedema. I'm continuously going to the hospital and doctor appointments, but I am strong!

REMINDER

Always remember to advocate for yourself, ask for help when needed, if your body feels different say something, document your days through treatments, ask for resources to help you through your journey and stay strong!

QUOTE

Some days she's a warrior. Some days she's a broken mess. Most days she's a bit of both. But everyday she's there. Standing. Fighting. Trying.

WORKING MY WAY BACK TO ME

BY CARA

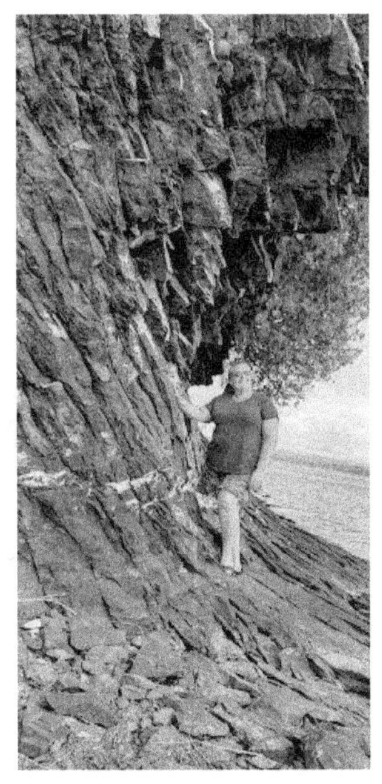

My cancer story starts a year before I was diagnosed. In June of 2021 I went for my yearly mammogram and was called back for more images. I was told I had a benign cyst measuring 3 cm and not to worry about it, that these things rarely ever turned into cancer. They told me it could get bigger and that if it bothered me they could remove fluid from it but otherwise it was fine. I was told I was good for another year for my mammogram. They also knew I have a family history of breast cancer, so I assumed they had taken that into consideration.

The cyst did get bigger, but I remembered the doctor's words so I did not worry about it. The cyst didn't hurt so I didn't call to have any fluid removed. A year went by and I went to have my mammogram done (June 2022). I was once again called back for more pictures and ultrasound which didn't surprise me as I already knew the cyst has gotten bigger. The images were suspicious, so I had to have a biopsy done.

In July of 2022 the test results came back. They made it to my patient portal account before the surgeon could call me so I opened them. I read the words "invasive ductal carcinoma" and the air was sucked out of my lungs. I would have collapsed on the kitchen floor if I had not grabbed the edge of the island. My legs were shaky and weak and the room was spinning. I called my husband to come home and told him about the results. I was a complete mess, wondering what was going to happen to me, was I going to lose my breast or worse, was I going die? The surgeon called me about 15 minutes after I read the results and talked to me about the results and options. It was so much to take in all at once and I was so shocked that nothing really stuck in my head. I had to call the surgeon back the next day to talk about it more. Ironically, the day I found out I had cancer was the day I went to the salon and donated 14" of my gorgeously thick hair to an organization that makes wigs for children undergoing cancer treatment.

After consulting with the surgeon and the oncology doctors I chose to do a lumpectomy, chemotherapy, and then radiation.

I want to point out that I've included the misdiagnosis because a lesson I learned is not to trust the doctors you are dealing with to take all things into consideration, and that if you feel something is not right, say something. I had the right to demand that they either do a biopsy on that 3cm cyst, have it removed, or request I have a repeat visit in three or six months to check on the cyst. I did not do that because I trusted what the doctor said. I know he did not do this to hurt me or because he didn't care, but in the future, I will not let concerning results go unchecked. If I had advocated for myself and demanded more be done, I might have saved myself some pain and suffering, not to mention exposure to the extremely strong treatments that have long term side effects.

I chose to cut my hair short before I started chemo. I figured it would make it easier for me to shave it when it started falling out and give me a little control over what was happening.

My lumpectomy surgery was done in August and then a port was surgically placed on September 27th. I started chemo September 30th. I had four treatments with two different drugs each time. I tolerated it well with the anti-nausea medication they gave before the treatments, and I felt pretty good with the steroids I had to take just before and after treatment. I could not eat however, because the treatments triggered diverticulitis attacks pretty much every time. I had to be on a liquid diet just before and for several days after each treatment. I finished chemo on December 2nd. Once the medication was out of my GI system and I was feeling better I was able to eat normally again. After the second treatment, my hair started falling out and I shaved it a few days later. Not having any hair was really hard for me. I loved my long, thick hair and I got a lot of compliments on it. It was one of my favorite things about me physically. I chose to wear wigs but also wore caps frequently.

I started radiation treatment January 4th and finished February 9th. Radiation was a lot easier but toward the end I was getting very tired. I had also gained a bunch of weight which didn't help.

My husband and I had been planning to go to Florida that winter, so once I had my follow up appointment after radiation, we took off and stayed down there for two weeks. It was so nice to get away, I needed it so bad after everything that happened. We rented a nice ranch house, and I went out to visit the farm animals every day and collect the eggs. They had sheep, donkeys, chickens, a horse and a few cows. Near the end of our stay, we met the owners who were really nice.

Fast forward to today. I am significantly overweight, and I am tired all the time. It hasn't been that long since I've completed treatment (less than a year). I've been struggling with different hormone therapies. Anastrozole made my hands hurt so bad that I could hardly use them to open jars and do much of anything, even write and sign my name or crochet. After several months of not being on the medication my hands are almost back to normal.

The next medication made my fatigue even worse, so I took a break from it. After consulting with my oncologist, I am going to try it again because the other medications are almost the same as Anastrozole and the only other one is Tamoxifen which has more serious side effects (even if rare, I didn't want to take the chance unless nothing else works). As part of my recovery, I am working on eating more protein with fruits and veggies, exercising, and working on shifting my mindset from "survivor" to "thriver". I have been really depressed lately and feel as if I will not be able to lose all the weight and that I'll never get my energy back. I am challenging myself to change that way of thinking and take better care of myself. I used to be so active and did lots of fun things like kayaking, paddleboarding, swimming, snowshoeing, running 5Ks and other adventurous things. I miss doing all these things and having the energy and confidence to do them.

Now I don't recognize myself in the mirror and I don't feel like myself at all. My body is extremely round where it used to be curvy, and my hair came back extremely curly and is still very curly almost a year later. I am looking forward to when it's long enough to put it up. One thing I have learned from all of this is that I can do hard things. Even though I was so scared of everything that was happening to me I showed up for the surgeries, the treatments, the blood work, all the needle sticks (truly hard for someone who is needle phobic) and I came out the other side a changed person in many ways. Some good and some not so good.

Time to start working my way back to me. I know I won't be exactly as I was before; I am forever changed, but I want to get back to feeling more like myself and I need to have energy to do some of the things I love.

10

NORMAL? WHAT'S THAT?

BY PATRICIA GREENE

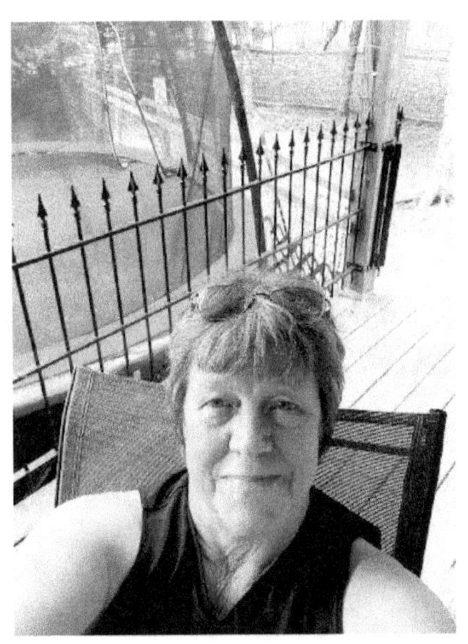

In 1997, I hit 40 and decided to have my first mammogram. I went to my gyn for my routine checkup and asked him about getting one. He told me I didn't need to worry about it, that my breasts were so small that I should not have any problem detecting anything abnormal. His nurse disagreed and chimed in with: "She should at least have one for a baseline."

It was almost another year before I finally got my first mammogram, and it was fine. I was thankful for the baseline.

I was always consistent about going every year for my annual "female" checkup. As much as I hated it, I knew it was one those "must do" checkups on my list.

Later in 1998, I went for my routine checkup, but this time I had a bad pap test. I had to go in for a biopsy. I was a complete mess. I had just been diagnosed with Von Willebrands Disease in 1996, which just seemed to complicate my life and any decision I had to make about any type of surgery. (Von Willebrands is a blood clotting disorder, a factor eight deficiency). Since this was my first surgery since I was diagnosed with this condition, I had no idea what I needed to do.

Living in a small community there wasn't a whole lot of doctors who specialized in this disorder. I felt lost. I went to my family doctor, and he told me that he really did not know much about it, and that the best thing to do was to go to the library and look it up. Of course, the internet was a much better tool to use, even if it was dial up!

The only doctor we had nearby who knew anything about this disorder was a local oncologist/hematologist. I went to see him for advice He looked at me and asked me:

"Why are you so freaked out about the biopsy? Are you afraid you have cancer?"

I was taken back by his lack of compassion and his reaction to my upcoming procedure.

I said, "Yes!"

He didn't offer any specific recommendations for how to handle Von Willebrands with regard to surgery. I had the biopsy, without any precautions. It was outpatient surgery, and I was assured it was not a big deal and I would be okay.

I ended up bleeding extensively. I honestly thought I was bleeding to death. I could not walk across the floor without having to sit down and rest. My legs felt like I had weights tied to them. I finally gave up and called my family doctor. Dr. C, and he sent me to the hospital asap for blood work. He put me on bedrest, no work, no lifting.

When I got my results back from my biopsy it showed precancerous cells, and I would need another surgery to remove them. I thought "OH Great!"

Many things happened that should have not happened. And it is a long story, But I will say this, when my test came back and I needed more surgery, I went to the city and searched out a physician/Hematologist who had a better handle on Von Willebrands disease. I had surgery at Magee's Womens' Hospital in Pittsburgh, PA. It was so scary, the thought of having the big C word.

I had the surgery, a cervical LEEP,. They removed the top layer of tissue from your cervix, which removes the cancerous cell. I had to spend the 2 nights to make sure I wasn't going to have any complications. I did really well with the surgery! Because I had all the right treatment in place.

I switched my doctor to a female doctor, Paulette, who was my guiding light, and I am so thankful for her. She insisted on me getting a mammogram and did all the routine work up I needed done. She was like a breath of fresh air for me. She supported me and took the time to find out more about what VWB was and what I needed to know.

In 1999 during a routine mammogram, I had my first "OH sh*t" moment. My mammogram showed a cluster of micro calcifications in my left breast. Here we go again… I had the biopsy here in town, with a local surgeon, Dr. J. Everything went rather well, he went in and scooped out the cluster and the pathology test came back and I was good to go.

Until……….

I hit menopause, or should I say, it hit me like a freight train! The hot flashes were so bad. I would have them all day and all night long. The brain fog, the weight gain, the bloating, irritable, oh and the mood swings! My poor family. I was exhausted all the time, which makes you even more cranky than normal.

I started to take an over the counter drug made for women who are going through menopause. I would take the daytime one and the nighttime one. Anything I could do for relief. I had so much happening in my life at that time I couldn't afford to feel this way! I had just become a grandma for the first time, and I had met the man I would eventually marry. I had just Graduated PennState, I was enjoying life; I was the happiest I had been in a very long time. So, I had no time or room to feel as crazy as menopause can make you feel.

In 2009 I started having some issues with my left breast. I thought maybe it was scar tissue or something from the biopsy I had years before. I made an appointment with Paulette and explained that my breast itched so badly all the time, no matter what I did I could not stop the itching; it was a deep itch that you couldn't satisfy. I told her I felt like I wanted to pull my nipple right off my body! She gave me some cream to see if that would help. I also told her about the OTC drug I was taking for the hot flashes and menopause. She warned me that the over-the-counter drug I was taking was linked to breast cancer and I should be very careful. I was shocked, if it was linked to breast cancer why can they advertise it the way they do and sell it over the counter?

In January 2010, it was time for my routine checkup with her. Paulette would have you do the mammogram first and then come for your visit. Later that day she called me and told me that I would need an ultrasound, for me not to get upset but they found something that needed more testing. I was not too alarmed, I figured it was no big deal. I went in 2 days later for the ultrasound. I saw the lump, still thinking it was no big deal, but not surprised it was in my nipple where all the itching was! My doctor called me later that day and told me that I needed a biopsy. Great… we were just moving into our new home. We were looking forward to it so much.

As luck had it, I had just made an appointment with our new surgeon, Dr. F. I had some other things that needed taken care of, so I already had an appointment to see her the next day. Paulette sent her everything and the biopsy was scheduled for the following week. I was to have the needle biopsy. I have issues with Novocain so she used lidocaine. BAD idea, I felt the whole thing. She asked me if I wanted her to stop, I told her "No, we are this far just keep going". It was only a couple of days when she got back to me. The doctor told me that they needed a bigger sample. Dr. F had put me on the schedule already. I had the biopsy, and the worst part started… the waiting!

A week later I was lying in bed all snuggled up with my (now ex) husband watching the snowfall. We were having the worst snowstorm; it was falling so fast. It was those big flakes that don't take long to pile up. The phone rang, it was the doctor's office. She wanted me to come in. I told her I didn't know if we could get out, could she just talk to me on the phone? She told me no, that I needed to come in. I was trembling, I knew if she wanted to see me in person that it wasn't good news. I looked at my husband with tears in my eyes. He hugged me and just held me.

He said, "I will have to put the chains on the truck, we will be okay."

I called my daughter at work, and I was in tears. She told me she would meet me at the doctor's office, I told her "The roads are too bad, don't risk it!" But she said, "I will meet you there!"

We all got there and I was a nervous wreck, they called us into the exam room and she opened up my file.

"Your test came back positive, you have cancer" everything after that was a blur. The air in the room was sucked out, my ears were ringing, and my head was buzzing. She went on to explain that I needed an MRI to see what was going on, and that my margins were too close, and she recommended a mastectomy. I had ductal carcinoma in situ*, as well as lobular carcinoma in situ*, the difference being the *DCIS* is cancer, and LCIS is precancerous. I didn't know the right questions to ask at the time. I was numb. She told me that MRI was waiting for me, and we would talk later. The rest of

that day is hazy. We came home and I was in shock. I don't know what I would have done without Craig by my side. I was a total mess. I believe I made a few phone calls and cried a lot.

The fear moved in and I thought I was going to die, I thought about all the treatments ahead, I thought about my grandchildren, my husband. What was I going to do? When that fear gets ahold of you, it turns into pure panic. I was in panic mode. I didn't sleep, I could hardly eat, my family did everything they could to help me keep busy so I wouldn't think about it. But it was all I could think about. I wanted it out of me and I wanted it out RIGHT NOW. I would sit up most of the night online looking stuff up and talking to other women. I eventually had a classmate reached out to me (Karen); she was such a tremendous comfort. She told me what to expect and reassured me that I would get through it. I was so thankful for her. I eventually learned there were more of my classmates and friends who went through this as they reached out to me. What an amazing support system!

Once all the tests were in, we made plans to move ahead with the mastectomy. My husband and I went to see a surgeon at Hillman Cancer Center in Pittsburgh, Dr E. He immediately put our fears to rest. I was so grateful for this man! The whole staff was amazing, kind and caring. We would become very close friends, I had no idea I was going to a regular. I talked to him about maybe having a double mastectomy, he told me he didn't feel the need for that, but if

I wanted one, he would do it. However, he explained "You have never had any issues with the other breast, so I think you will be okay." We discussed reconstruction there were so many choices. Turned out I did not have much of a choice. I went with the implants. I also opted out of the double and went with the single mastectomy.

I remember one day sitting alone in our den-office, I had my feet propped up and I was staring out the window. I was thinking about my beautiful grandchildren, my husband and our new home. I was feeling so full of gratitude and I said "God, what is going on here? I am finally happy, I have all the things I have wished for all my life, why is this happening to me now?" I was thinking about the garden I wanted to plant with my husband and I was thinking about Joely, my granddaughter. How much she loved being here with us. We would always plant lots of peas and we would snack on them as soon as they came up. She would always make sure to pick some for "papa". I again, said "God, what is going on?" as the tears rolled down my cheek and my heart was so heavy, I heard, "Everything will be okay" and my heart was full of peace and so full of love. And I knew.. "Be still and Know I am God" Psalms 46.10. So often we can't be still and listen. This was one of those moments. Yes, I was still worried, but I knew I was going to be ok.

My surgery was planned for April 15, 2010. My sister and her husband went with us the night before. We stayed in the family house in Pittsburgh. We went out to eat and tried to keep busy.

Surgery day, I was looking forward to getting this beast out of me, yet so traumatized by the fact I was losing a breast. I would have expanders put in place during my surgery and once I healed up, the process of filling the expanders would start. The day of the surgery was a whirlwind, we got to the hospital early and I had to have some test done. Then the blue dye is injected so they can trace your nodes. We were taken to a big waiting room with lots of other people all waiting for surgery. Craig was given a buzzer and a number so he could follow my surgery. They finally called my name and I had to go alone to a private waiting area where I would be prepped for surgery. I had to receive my medicine for my bleeding disorder, and that was another process. I was a mess and I kept asking to please, please, let my husband come in with me. Finally, they went and got him. He was my rock and I was so glad he was there.

Finally, it was my turn to go. He gave me a kiss and off I went. I remember being wheeled into the cold room and moving on to the bed. There were so many people in there and each one of them introduced themselves and told me what their job was. It was time.. and I drifted off to sleep.

The next thing I remember is waking up as they were pushing me into my room, Craig was in the hall waiting for me with a big Thumbs up, meaning they got everything! My sister Carol, and her husband Phil were also there. I looked down and I noticed my breast was gone. Then I drifted back off to sleep.

Dr E had put the expander in and it felt like a really tight bra that couldn't be removed. I was very uncomfortable. I kept telling myself I would get use to it, just give it time. And those drain tubes were a NIGHTMARE. I stayed a few days and then I was ready to come home. Yes, I did a lot of crying during that time. I was sad and relieved, and angry, most of all I felt betrayed by my body. I was an emotional mess.

At home, Craig would come home every day at lunchtime and take care of my drains. That probably was one of the worst things to deal with. They were so sore, and I just couldn't do it myself. I had the drains in a lot longer than most people did, 3 long weeks. I am sure it was because of my VWD. I couldn't wait to get them out!

After the healing,(5 months) I started the process of filling my expanders. Craig went with me the first time since we had no idea what to expect. But after that I would drive to Pittsburg (3 hours one way) every week, see my doctor, and then drive back home. Sometimes my friend Marsha would go with me, but I mostly went alone. Many times, I would cry the whole way home, feeling so alone in this process. It made for a very long day.

Finally, the day came to swap out that awful expander and get my implant. I could not wait. I can't say I was disappointed with my implant, but it was odd. I didn't like the way it felt.

I was adjusting to my "new" look and trying to "fake" that everything was ok. After all, I was lucky (as I was told over and over) that they found it in time. I didn't feel very lucky. So many comments people made with good intentions, and I would never want any of them to feel bad about it. But telling someone they are lucky they had breast cancer, or any cancer, is something you just shouldn't say.

I had to go for a mammogram every 3 months for the other breast. Then it switched to 6 months. My first 6-month mammogram fell on the same day they had found the cancer before. I canceled it due to being superstitious and rescheduled if for the next month. And low and behold, it didn't matter! They found 2 spots that caused them some concern. So, off to Pittsburgh we went again for a biopsy. I had it done on Feb 18, 2011. Laying in that MRI-guided machine for 2 ½ hours was hard! My back hurt, my body hurt! I finally asked the doctor how much longer was it going to be? She told me that there were more than 2 spots, she said there was 6. I said, "You are not going to have to biopsy all of them, are you?" She reassured me that was not the case.

I thought that if it took 2 hours to do the first 2, I would be in that machine for another 2 hours. The staff reassured me that I was almost done. Define "almost" please? Another 30 minutes went by, I said jokingly, "My Ativan is going to wear off soon, so I hope we are almost done." I was told that they were almost done(again), and then the doctor explained to me what was going on. It was taking so long, because apparently the one spot they were most concerned about was right up against my chest wall and was a little harder to get to.

Finally, I was free! They patched me up, told me not to drive for 24 hours, and I would hear from my doctor soon.

We got home around 6 that night and my daughter called me and told me that Gram (my mother) wasn't doing well, and I should go see her right now. Mom had gotten sick about 6 months prior and I had to put her in a nursing home. She was suffering from Dementia. So, Craig took me over to see what was going on. She was out of it. I sat with her for a little while, but she asked me where I was, and I didn't want to alarm her. I didn't tell her. She was very much aware I was there and who I was.. She kept telling me she was "dying", she felt she was over medicated. I had the nurse print out all her medications and I told mom I would call the doctor first thing on Monday.

Sunday February 20, 2011 I got a phone call at 9 am saying they were taking mom to the hospital and that I should get there as soon as possible. I got dressed, called my sister and ran out the door. I met mom as they were taking her upstairs to ICU. It broke my heart to see her like this. She had always been so strong and now she was just lying there, eyes sunken, and the look of confusion on her face. She saw me and right away,

She said "Patty, thank God you're here."

Those were the last words my mother ever spoke to me.

I hurried and called all my kids to come and see her. We were all around her talking about all the funny things she did. I told her how much I loved her and then I prayed for Jesus to come and take her home. Not 10 minutes later, she was gone.

The next day my sister and I were making funeral arrangements when I got a phone call from Craig. He said the doctor called and they needed me to call them back. I called them back and they told me that the spots were "atypical" and that they needed to take bigger samples. We talked a little bit, and I made the decision to just have them take the other breast.

I said, "Let me finish the funeral arrangements for my mother and we will get it done. Then we are done, I don't have a third one!"

Two weeks later I was under the knife having my right breast removed. It was 11 month almost to the day of my first surgery. I found out after all was said and done, the mastectomy was a very smart decision. I am glad I did what I did.

I had him put the expander in for my implant, and I started five months later getting my fills. Another six months of driving back and forth to Pittsburgh.

I had my implants for 10 years, and I hated almost every minute of it. I had the left one replaced four times and the right one twice. I slept in a recliner most of the time because lying flat felt like I had bricks on my chest and made it hard to breath. They were hard and I felt like I was having muscle spasms in the left one all the time. My lymph nodes would swell up and make my arm pits hurt. I was sick all the time. I was stressed out all the time. My blood pressure was high, I developed COPD, I had a rash from my thighs down that itched and was red and prickly. The worse was the brain fog and the weight gain. I seemed to function well enough to fool everyone else, but I was a mess. I had been on one heck of an emotional roller coaster and I wanted off.

After more surgeries and biopsies then I can count, I had enough. I decided to have them removed and go flat. My husband agreed with me and assured me it didn't matter to him, so I went ahead with the removals.

January 2020, right before Covid hit, I had my implants removed.

Immediately the brain fog was GONE, and the rash disappeared in 2 weeks. I could lay flat on my belly again. I started to lose weight. I felt so much better. Now, I cannot say that it was for sure getting the implants out, but I can only tell you how I felt right away.

I miss my real breasts, but I do not miss those two things that hung on my chest and pretended to be breasts. Having breasts or not did not make me more or less of a woman. Some women get them and have no problems with them. I was not one of them. Again, I made the right choice for me and I have no regrets. It was an emotional decision to get the implants. I thought it would make me feel "normal." I thought also about my husband and I was only 52 at the time. Instead of making me feel normal, they did the opposite, I felt fake. Being flat isn't the worst thing. I never was big chested anyway. I am still adjusting. I am finding my new "Normal".

You never know what a person is going through. That is why it is so important to treat each other with kindness and compassion. It could make a difference that could change lives.

Unfortunately, Craig and I split up a year after I had my implants removed. I am grateful that he was with me during those hard times. I think there was just so much damage done to our relationship over the years. I got breast cancer back to back, lost my mother and then lost my son all in the matter of 4 years. It was a very hard time for me. It played on me emotionally and physically. I felt broken.

Everything that has happened in my life has taught me some kind of lesson. So yes, I am lucky and I am blessed.

I have learned to speak up for myself and I don't just go with the flow. I have had some real battles. I have had medical professionals try to make me feel like I did not know what I was talking about or that I didn't know my own body. I stood my ground and if I wouldn't have, who knows what could have happened. Don't be afraid to ask questions, don't be afraid to say "no" if something doesn't feel right. Do not be afraid to get a second opinion if you don't agree, or a third one, or a fourth one. Do whatever it takes until YOU feel right about it. Don't let anyone tell you different or make you feel wrong for wanting another opinion. This is our battle, we are the ones that have to live with the decisions we make. We did not ask for this, but we do get to choose how we react to it. And most of all, be kind to yourself. One thing I have learned through all of this is to be true to yourself, always.

FYI

Reference

Ductal carcinoma in situ (DCIS) is a condition that affects the cells of the milk ducts in the breast. The cells lining the milk ducts turn malignant (cancerous) but stay in place (in situ). DCIS is an early form of breast cancer.
https://www.hopkinsmedicine.org/

Lobular carcinoma in situ (LCIS) means abnormal cells are in the breast. *LCIS* is not cancer but can signal a higher risk of *breast cancer.*
American Cancer Society

Von Willebrand Disease is a lifelong bleeding disorder in which your blood doesn't clot properly. People with the disease have low levels of von Willebrand factor, a protein that helps blood clot, or the protein doesn't perform as it should.
https://www.mayoclinic.org

MRI Guided Core Needle Biopsy- Breast Imaging
It is performed to evaluate a suspicious finding seen on a **breast MRI**. It is completed on an outpatient basis with minimal discomfort and recovery time.
https://www.uclahealth.org

****my breast cancer was estrogen fed.***

Microcalcifications: *These show up as fine, white specks, similar to grains of salt. They're usually noncancerous, but certain patterns can be an early sign of cancer.*
https://www.mayoclinic.org/

11

FROM A THORN TO A SWORD IN MY DNA

BY DAWN FARMER*

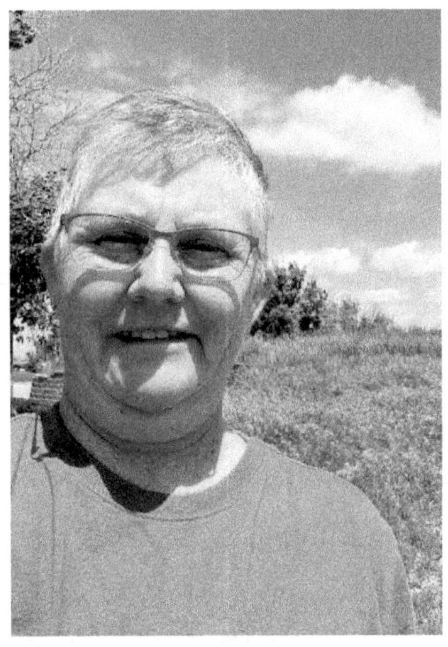

Growing up, cancer was never really on my radar. My grandparents had died from all sorts of other things like a heart attack, emphysema, a car accident, and congestive heart failure. I can't even recall anyone I know who had cancer or went through chemotherapy. So in June of 1992 when my mom came for a visit and was struggling with bad leg lymphedema, we weren't sure what to expect. Some scans and an ultrasound quickly confirmed cancer. A soft tumor the size of a softball filled her abdomen and originated from her ovary. They couldn't feel it, but when she had surgery, it was spread beyond what they could even attempt to remove. She didn't fit the "typical" signs of those with ovarian cancer, as she ate a healthy, low meat, high plant diet, exercised, and was at an ideal weight and all. She survived until December of that year. I was 24 years old.

Growing up, I was raised with lots of moves and time spent overseas. I had never lived in any place longer than 4 years when I went to college in a small rural town in Indiana. I met my husband (Tom) there, and we married after we graduated from college in 1990. We were young, pursuing our careers, and had just bought a small starter house in Muncie, Indiana. I was completing the student teaching portion of a teaching degree in Biology and general science for middle school and high school. My husband was also a teacher by training, but unable to find a teaching job he ended up working as a computer support technician. After a bit, I began to pursue my Master's Degree in Biology with an emphasis on plants, and Tom continued to work with computers. After completing my research, I began to teach high school and middle school while working on my thesis.

As a Biology teacher, I was always interested in new things that were occurring in the science field. I remember the news when they first identified a gene that when mutated could cause cancer, p53. This was the first time we could pinpoint that certain genes regulated DNA and when they failed, cells with damaged DNA resulted and they could cause cancer. I found this fascinating and had discussions with students about the potential genetic revolution that was happening in the early 1990's. It was radical thinking about the possibilities that might open up as we better understood the potential and promise of genetics.

In 1996 we moved out into the country into a small home on 24 acres. We were thrilled to be out of town, on some land, and thinking about the possibilities and promise of land. My husband had switched where he was working but was still in Information Technology. He began to work on a Master's Degree, which he completed in 1998. We also welcomed our first son in May 1997. We were thrilled. We both worked hard in our respective jobs and in June 1999 welcomed our 2nd son. After finishing his Master's Degree, Tom was able to switch jobs, and with his new position, I was able to stay home, where I completed the written work for my Master's Thesis, and soon baby 3 was on its way. I graduated with a MS in December 2000, and in July 2001 we welcomed son number 3. These were busy, but good years. I began to grow a garden and that soon morphed into selling produce and garden vegetable starts. We also began to raise beef cattle as with a growing family we wanted to be able to provide our family with healthy and clean foods.

Tom and I experienced a heartbreaker, when what we hoped would be our 4th child, ended in a miscarriage. This was stressful and Tom ended up with a bad case of shingles. Shortly after that, we were expecting again and this would turn out to be our 4th child, which would complete our family. We were elated when he arrived in November 2003. We were done having children, but very happy with our crew of 4 guys.

I had gone in for annual skin exams for several years and it was not uncommon to have spots removed but they had always been benign or precancerous. Having lived overseas in the tropics and California when I was growing up, I had been exposed to lots of tropical sun, too many sunburns to count, and was pretty high risk for skin cancer. This exam in 2005, was routine, other than when I pointed out a spot that had seemed of late to be growing bigger, getting darker and irregular. The dermatologist did a quick biopsy and sent me out the door. I had other biopsies, and didn't think too much of this, when I didn't get a letter with the results, I called. It's never a good thing when they won't tell you the info over the phone, but set up an office visit. So in short order, I was scheduled with a surgeon to remove a silver dollar-sized spot on my forearm. Thankfully we had caught the Melanoma in stage 0. It was very early and I escaped with just surgery as there were clear margins. No chemo, no radiation, but pretty quick recovery of the railroad track on my arm. Up to this point, I had been very careful to help my children avoid sunburns, but after this, I was even more dogmatic that they wear hats and sunscreen, avoid peak UV hours, and avoid sunburns. I would do my best to protect them.

In early 2006, my maternal Aunt called and let us know she had breast cancer. This call, made us sit up and take notice. Because of my mother's ovarian cancer and her breast cancer, the doctor recommended a genetic test to see if there was a chance that our family carried a cancer-causing mutated gene. Genetic research had undergone massive growth and a huge increase in knowledge and options. When the results came back, she was BRCA2 positive, and it was likely that my mother would have been also. I did what research I could and determined that I wanted to be tested so that I could approach my future with the most knowledge possible. This was before Obamacare, and there was a fear that if my genetics test came back BRCA2 posi-tive, the insurance would not cover any treatments as my cancer would be a pre-existing condition. In light of this, we paid for the test out of pocket using our tax refund for the year and did not send the results to the insurance company.

When we sat down with the genetics counselor, I was surprised to learn that I was not BRCA2 positive. This surprised me because melanoma is a common cancer in people with BRCA2. I gave this information to my dermatologist and my general practitioner.

It was not enough that I knew, I had siblings, as well as cousins, who could also be carriers of the gene, and be at an increased risk of cancer also. I drafted up a letter explaining the test, and the options from low to high, and got permission from my Aunt to include her results as well as several informative guides with best practice at the time. I mailed this package to my siblings and my cousins and heard crickets. I knew about genetic cancer, and their potential risk of getting it, and wanted them to be informed. I had hoped for more conversations and was willing to answer questions or point to further resources.

Life continued on for a couple of years, our cattle herd continued to slowly expand, and greenhouses were added for produce and garden starts. We were able to move into a larger home across the road, and we kept our small home for renters because we were using the land to farm. The house we moved out of was tiny and our growing boys needed more space. During this time, cancer hit close again. A teacher of several of my sons (different times), came down with breast cancer. She continued to teach as she went through treatment, which resulted in her losing her hair. Knowing that the teacher was having her hair shaved off before it all fell out, the mothers of kids in her class (who had the same hairdresser), arranged for the boys in the class to all meet with the teacher's hairdresser who shaved all their heads so that they would be in solidarity with the teacher. So the day she came in with a wig on, the boys all walked into class with hats on and then pulled them off. She and I had several conversations as she was also dealing with a genetics-based cancer.

As all my boys were now in school, I began to sub at the school where they went. It was a K-12 school so they were all in the same building. I ended up teaching Spanish for three years until I was going to have to go back to school to get certified in Spanish to continue. I really didn't have a desire to return for more schooling when I had a Master's in Biology. So I stepped back and stayed on the farm, for a bit. We had also begun to raise Anatolian Shepherd livestock guardian dogs. So between the cattle, greenhouses, and dogs, I had quite a bit to keep me busy. This went on for a year until I got a call from another school asking if I was willing to teach science. Since my oldest was now able to drive, and could take his brothers to school, I took the job.

The year 2016 began most like others, but my husband and I just had an unsettled feeling. I can't explain it, but it was as if our intuition was letting us know, a big change was coming. It was also a very difficult year as my husband's dad was not able to fight off pneumonia, and sadly passed away. Things at Tom's work took a turn for the worse when a new President came in and began to replace the top-level leadership, including director-level positions, throughout the organization. Tom began looking for a new job and filled out application after application for jobs he was qualified for. He got nothing but silence. That was so frustrating. At this point, we also began to shut down the farm. We sold off our cattle herd in different groups, and we began to sell equipment.

Tom then began a wider search for a job more similar to what he was currently doing in 2017. He got an interview in Scranton, PA. This would be a major move to an area where we didn't know anyone and didn't have any family nearby. He was offered a position and we agreed that it seemed the best option at the time, and he began his new work in December. This meant I was at home with 3 sons, a HS senior (finalizing college applications, plans, and such), a HS junior, and an 8th grader. Our oldest son was in college in Michigan. This was the first time in our marriage that we were apart for an extended period. He would work long hours during the week, and then for one extended weekend a month Tom would drive back to Indiana to see the kids and spend some time at home. We were also packing and each time he returned to Pennsylvania, he would take a load of things back with him in a progressive move. This was a really hard time for me as I was in charge of what was left of the farm (45 acres), selling the last equipment, kids, a graduation party planning, teaching, and packing to boot. I had my annual mammogram in March 2018 which came back clear. I started mammograms early and had them regularly because of my family history.

This high-stress time in our lives was only put on steroids when one afternoon the school administration walked down to my classroom and called me out into the hallway. My oldest son who was away at college had a non-fatal suicide attempt and was in the psychiatric ward at a hospital in Michigan where he attended college. For a moment my world went blank. They told me I could walk out right then and they would cover, but my mind needed to think a little, and it sounds crazy, but I went back in and finished the lesson and scratched out rudimentary lesson plans for the next couple of days. I also called my husband and we formulated a plan. He was in Pennsylvania and it would take him a much longer time to arrive and I wanted to go and see my son. I went home grabbed a few items and headed to my other kids' school. I pulled them all out of class and explained what had happened with their brother, that I needed to go to Michigan and that dad was on his way home and would be there that evening. This was causing stress hormones to flood through my veins. My 2nd oldest son could drive the other boys home as usual, could fix dinner, and their dad would be home before too late that evening.

I put the truck in D and headed up to Michigan. I was grateful my son was alive, but it was only because of the action of a friend who called for help after a weird text from my son. We realized how close we were to not having a son. This was incredibly hard emotionally at any time, more so in the chaos of what was already going on. After a week of him in the hospital, and visits from my husband and I, we were able to bring him home and collect his stuff from college. We were going to move to Pennsylvania so we didn't feel it smart to get him started with a mental health professional in Indiana and then move, and restart in Pennsylvania. This brought on an entirely new set of fears. While he was on some meds, would I come home to find him alive or not daily? We made it through the end of the school year, graduation, and the graduation party, and thankfully we were all there as a family.

During this time, my husband was finally able to purchase a home for us in Pennsylvania, moving out of the rental he was in, so there would be a place for us to land when we arrived. At the end of May, my oldest and my 3rd son moved to Pennsylvania with their dad, after school was out. I went hard at painting, finishing up projects, maintaining yards, and getting 2 properties and homes for sale. Throughout June, we moved the other two sons and more stuff out to Pennsylvania, so by July, I was left by myself with only what I needed to eat, sleep, maintain the yard, and do repairs. The big house sold, and we closed in August. Now I was the one making trips out to PA to see my family, and pets and heading back to Indiana to keep working. One day, I had the weirdest sensation. It was like an electric shock without quite the pain in my left breast. It happened 2x in quick succession and then never again. It didn't feel like a pulled muscle just kinda tingly.

Then one day, I got a long text from one of my sisters. She had just been diagnosed with stage IV ovarian cancer. This was a gut punch. I had earlier told my siblings about our risk but was now finding out that all 3 sisters were BRCA2 positive. My oldest sister chose to take preventive surgeries to reduce her risk, but the other two didn't do anything at that time.

In the midst of the crazy of what my sister told me, the second property contract was signed and the closing was set for early December. It had been a long summer, painting, flooring, cleaning barns, doing repairs, and maintaining everything, but I was so ready to get back to family full-time and let this chapter close. Life was still complicated as we were trying to help my third son with college applications, my youngest son was angry about moving to Pennsylvania to a much bigger school and gave us all kinds of grief for making him leave Indiana and his school. We were finally able to get a counselor, and doctor for my oldest son.

After Thanksgiving with family in late November, I did a breast self-exam and the internal structures just felt larger or thicker on my left side, no mass in particular, but just felt "different". So now I was in Pennsylvania, and I don't have a doctor, I don't know any doctors, and I have no idea where to start. My husband sent out an email to his female colleagues, and all 3 of them responded that they used the same Dr., and liked her as their General Practitioner. So this was a place to start. Her office was taking applications online and I filled one out. They took my concerns seriously and I was quickly able to get a doctor's visit on December 3rd, 2018. The doctor listened to my family history of cancer and set me up for every possible cancer check you can reasonably do. So I had a date for a 3-D mammogram and ultrasound, dermatologist, Ob-Gyn, optometrist, and Colonoscopy all within a month. It was hard enough to be new to the area, but this would make your head spin. I drove back to Indiana for the house closing and was back in Pennsylvania for the appointment shortly after.

On December 10, 2018, I was sent for a Mammogram and Ultrasound. They found a small mass and recommended a biopsy. The doctor who did the biopsies was not there that day, and I was sent back on the 18th to complete the biopsy. I was not given enough pain meds and it was extremely painful. After the biopsy, clips were also placed and a follow-up mammogram was done. December 20th, my results came back as Invasive Mammary Lobular Cancer in the left breast, and the biopsied lymph node grade 1. What a crappy Christmas present. We didn't tell our sons what was going on until after Christmas, but with the next treatments coming up, they needed to know what was occurring and we wanted to be upfront and honest with them. Up until this point we had tried to hide what was going on. They suspected something, but not what we had to tell them.

The doctor's visits were non-stop for a bit. I met with an Oncologist, Radiologist, and also a Surgeon for port placement. January 2nd my port was placed and I was scheduled for a class on the upcoming chemotherapy that I would be facing. It was hard to process it all. Then before I started chemo, the oncologist found a discrepancy between my mammogram and ultrasound on the size of my tumor. She sent me in for a breast MRI to better determine what we were dealing with. I was set to start Chemotherapy on Jan 10th, but that was put on hold after my Oncologist got the MRI report back. She didn't like what she was seeing in my right breast. Now I needed to do an MRI biopsy, as the 3D Mammogram didn't pick up anything in my right breast, but the MRI did. This time I asked for extra numbing to be applied and it was a much less painful procedure. Three locations in my right breast were biopsied and an additional lymph node on the right side.

On January 17th the results came back that all areas biopsied in my right breast and lymph node came back positive for lobular cancer, and because of my family history the Oncologist ordered a genetics test. I explained that I had tested for BRCA2 and it was negative, but I wasn't sure what a new test would show.

Then thanks to my general practitioner, I was scheduled for a colonoscopy on January 21, and thankfully no polyps were found. The next day I started Chemotherapy. It started with 4 Adriomycin (Red Devil) and Cytoxan was given 2x a month for four rounds.

A week after my first chemotherapy, I was in the doctor's office for my second chemo when they let me know that my genetics test had come back. I did not have BRCA2, but I was a carrier for the NF1 gene. The oncologist had also asked for a PET scan when I was diagnosed earlier, but insurance denied the PET and I was left with a CT and a bone scan after having started chemotherapy. I still wonder if insurance would not have denied the PET scan if it might have shown my cancer had already spread at the beginning, you can only do what they will pay for. The CT and Bone scan showed some nodules in the lungs as well as sclerotic lesions in some of the thoracic spine, sternum, the right femoral neck that could be metastatic disease, but the spots were so small, the oncologist thought it best to continue aggressive treatments. At this point, I wished they had done the scans before beginning chemotherapy. Lobular cancer is more difficult to detect as does not form masses, but long stringy growth that is much harder to detect. If I knew then, what I know now, I would have demanded the PET as it was my best chance to see where the cancer was.

My hair began to fall out and we shaved it off on February 5th. It was cold, so a hat in the winter is not bad, but it is so weird that the stubs of hair that were left hurt if they touched things. I couldn't stand a hat, pillow, or anything touching my head. I had my husband take a razor and make my head smooth and completely devoid of hair. This was much more comfortable.

So I finished my Red Devil and Cytoxan and proceeded on to 12 doses of taxol, once weekly. I tolerated chemotherapy with mostly brain fog and lethargy, but thankfully no neuropathy. But chemotherapy took from Jan to May when I felt bad, didn't have lots of energy and as we found out later, didn't help as hoped.

I had a follow-up MRI and it showed a decrease in size of the tumors but persistent bilateral axillary lymph nodes with cortical thickening. There was some decrease, but not a complete resolution. Having completed chemotherapy, I was set up for a bilateral mastectomy on July 12th. I had researched my options and asked for Aesthetic Flat Closure as I was not going to do reconstruction and wanted to have a smooth chest and start to heal and move on. I took pictures in and was super clear with the surgeon. There was no doubt what I was asking for, in fact, I asked him to sign that he understood what I was asking for. He refused to sign, and that should have made me stand up and walk out of his office. But at this point, you are incredibly vulnerable. There is a power dynamic with them having the power, 100% control of the situation when you are under anesthesia and not much recourse.

After a two-and-a-half-day hospital stay, I was able to go home. After a few more days, I was able to remove the bandages. My poor husband was so careful and kind, but dang did it hurt. It took around 30 minutes and we were both just about in tears. The pain of removing the tape on a very sore body and then the double pain of being denied what I had asked and paid for. The surgeon left me with enough skin so that I could put expanders in and do reconstruction. This was a huge low point in my journey. I felt defeated, not listened to, and quite frankly abused. I was so furious when I had to go back for weekly checkups, a seroma draining, and then finally to have the drains removed. I asked him why he disregarded my wishes and he retorted "You can have a revision later." I was so pissed, I couldn't say anything more as I was afraid of what would come out of my mouth. He did what he wanted and took my money, instead of being honest and saying either 1)He wasn't capable of performing Aesthetic Flat Closure (AFC), or 2)bringing in a Plastic surgeon who could complete what I had asked for, but reducing how much he would make on the surgery. I also felt betrayed by the oncologist as I had trusted her to find a capable surgeon and she knew I wanted AFC with no reconstruction.

The pathology report from the mastectomy and lymph node dissection showed that the cancer was still in every lymph node (5 on one side and 7 on the other), that was examined and not completely resolved in my breasts. The neoadjuvant chemotherapy had not worked. My Oncologist then sent me to a different oncologist to see if there were any clinical studies that I could participate in. This Dr was very thorough in looking through my scans, recent pathology, and such. She noted that there were no studies currently, but she also explained that I was likely either stage 3 but highly likely stage 4 and she was sorry. In some ways, I felt my original oncologist knew I was stage IV, but wanted someone else to tell me. So she sent me on to the Radiologist which would be my next step after I healed from the double mastectomy.

When I met with the Radiologist, she was sorry about the surgery but wanted to get things set up for radiation. I asked her what was the point of radiation (a localized treatment) if my cancer was metastatic and already all over my body. I was going to have full chest radiation as I had bilateral cancer and cancer in lymph nodes on both sides as well. Her response was insurance won't cover treatment for Metastatic disease unless you can directly show the disease has spread. I didn't want radiation as it would put my body through a lot and really wouldn't help me, but it would have a big impact on my quality of life and the potential radiation I would need down the road if this was metastatic disease. On top of everything else that had gone wrong, this just seemed like another punch down. I was frustrated, but where do you turn?

In August, after the disappointing results of chemotherapy, and the previous CT showing some odd bone results, insurance finally approved a PET. The PET scan showed some uptake in the areas of the mastectomy, and lymph nodes in the chest and noted as the CT of small skeletal sclerosis spots up and down the lumbar spine, in ribs, pelvis, and sternum. My oncologist armed me with scans and sent me down to an orthopedic oncologist and surgeon. He examined my scans and was unsure if the spots were bone islands or metastatic disease. The only problem he noted was that the spots were too small to biopsy as they needed a spot at least 5mm and he couldn't find any spots that size in a location they could biopsy. Again, frustrated at facing a failure to be able to pursue the path that would be best for my longevity.

Unbeknownst to us, the orthopedic oncologist had forwarded my scans to another doctor who was able to locate one spot on my sacrum large enough to be able to biopsy. In the meantime, I had met with my Oncologist, who stated that without proof of metastatic disease, I should proceed on to radiation. She called the radiologist and they had an opening that afternoon. I had the initial forms constructed, tattoos placed and CT done to set up radiation. This was really hard and super frustrating. I was set to start radiation on Sept 5th, but I got a call from the Orthopedic Oncologist that he heard back from the doctor he sent the scans. I could have a bone biopsy done on September 16 to see if the breast cancer had moved into my bones. After the procedure which I anticipated to be much worse than it was, it was now waiting. On September 18th, the bone biopsy found that focal metastatic carcinoma was compatible with breast origin. This was the demonstration that indeed it was Metastatic Breast Cancer. At this point, I was sent to another Oncologist to see if there were any clinical studies that I could join. The doctor said none were open, but did call my oncologist and recommend a recently approved drug called Kisquali.

On October 22nd I started my new line of treatment with Ibrance, Lupron, Faslodex, and Xgeva. I was finally on meds that helped me with the current state of my body. So while we were doing the best for my body, my mind had been in a very dark place since my double mastectomy and realization I was metastatic. It just seemed that every diagnosis was a worse step down into the cancer dungeon. Then when you read the long-term survival rates of metastatic breast cancer patients, it is pretty scary. It was really hard to process this all.

One of the best things my husband and I did was to attend a conference in the fall of 2019 which was put on by Susan G. Komen of NY just for Metastatic Breast Cancer (MBC) patients. They had multiple specialists speak, covered new research into meds, and there were lots of people who were in my shoes present. When we arrived, we were given a name tag with a color that represented how long someone was alive with MBC. I was assuming I might have a year and extra lucky if maybe two years. At this conference, I met someone who was still alive 10 years out, and living with MBC. Granted that wasn't the average, but it gave me a tremendous amount of hope that maybe I would see my youngest graduate from high school. They also had doctors who told us all the new meds coming down the pipeline and that if you had to have this sucky disease, this was one of the best times with research, new drugs, and things moving towards helping people live longer and better with MBC. This began to help me feel like I had a future, maybe not as long, but hopefully longer than the 2-year average that statistics indicated people with MBC survived. I had almost made it a year and was responding well to treatments, and treatments were providing me with a good quality of life.

One of the things I had forced myself to do during cancer was to reach out to others since I was in a new area and didn't have friends or family. There was a fantastic little gym for cancer patients at the cancer center where an incredibly kind trainer, Abby, would devise an exercise regimen for you and whatever medical issues you were facing (balance, strengthening, stretching, etc). All the members of this gym were there because they currently had, or in the past had cancer. It was such a healing and affirming place, I can't overstate how beneficial it was along with the benefits of exercise on cancer. FORCE was another group that initially provided me with a phone peer-to-peer person to help me with my initial diagnosis. Terry would check in, answer questions, and just give me support. This was helpful because even though my sister had cancer, she wasn't in a place to help someone else. I also found a dear friend, Michele, who was a breast cancer survivor, whom I met by chance at an event for our kids. She took me under her wing, took me to chemo, was open about her story, incredibly helpful, and we had the same oncologist that we could grouse about. I also attended several support groups and found another friend, Paula who was a previvor, but incredibly kind and generous. These friends took me to chemo, brought meals after surgery, and were a huge help to me and my family. It is harder to make friends as an adult, but when you find welcoming people they are gems.

I also found some fantastic people in supporting groups such as Unite For Her, Bravehearts, and an MBC group that had meet-ups. Many cancer patients are the most wonderful people, in the shittiest club. Cancer has a way of making you focus on the important, living your best life now with what you have, being real with who you are, and helping to drop the false narrative that we have it all together,

Then came COVID towards the end of 2019. Having cancer was bad, having COVID hanging over everything was a double whammy worse. Since my meds lowered my immune system, I was quarantined in our house. I would go for walks, but not get together with friends, support groups stopped, exercise groups stopped, and life as we knew it came to a standstill. I was grateful I was at a point where I didn't require hospital care. It was difficult at best and mentally a struggle. Schools closed for my sons, so everyone was at home doing online courses. My husband would do the shopping and he was mostly working from home too. Life as we knew it came to a screeching halt. I would go in monthly for treatment. Mask before entering, then a temp and questionnaire, then spaced out in waiting rooms, blood work, then back to 2nd waiting room, and then taken to the exam room. Weighed, BP measured, lungs checked, and whisked off to a third location for shots. On a good day, I only came home with 5 band-aids on. Those days my port was cantankerous, and blood was drawn from my arm with a 6th band aid. I would try to walk after shots as they were in my bum, and walking helped to reduce their causing lumps and more painful problems. As time proceeded, I would walk with friends outside, but we still masked. It was mentally good to see people again, even if we were outside and not too close. That was a huge help.

I also talked to my oncologist about having a revision on my chest. She pushed me off initially saying wait a year and we will talk about it. At this point, I was stable and brought the subject up again. Shots were available for COVID-19, medical facilities were much less crowded, and operations for elective surgeries were again allowed. She sent me to a plastic surgeon. It was a super weird thing. While were waiting in the examination room my husband had to use the restroom, which often happens when you have to drive long distances to get to the doctor's appointment. After he came back into the room, we waited and waited. When the doctor and nurse finally came in, they were rushed in and acted all hurried and all. The surgeon seemed dismissive of my meds and told me I needed to get info to him about them. What my husband told me later is that when he went to the restroom, they were all standing around and chatting it up and talking, and took their time to come in late to the appointment with no regard to us. We felt very dismissed and I canceled any upcoming procedures. One of my friends had a revision following new tumor growth and was super happy with her plastic surgeon. We were able to get an appointment with him and he was very clear about what he could do and what the outcome would be and was very supportive of my decision. I didn't expect a miracle, but it was nice to have someone be honest as to the expected outcome and treat me as a person, not a paycheck. I had the surgery as an outpatient in March 2021 and was exceedingly pleased with the result. My chest is clean, with no dog ears, and no extra tissue, and before the revision, I would occasionally have swelling under my armpits on my chest that no longer occurs as he removed extra skin. I am so much happier with the revision and just wish I would have had this Plastic surgeon with an actual breast surgeon the first time around and been able to have only one surgery instead of the expense, pain, and downtime from 2 surgeries. I recovered well and continued to respond to treatment well.

In May we had another life-shaking event. The place where my husband was working decided to outsource his department. Three months later the new company let my husband go and we were left with little to no income. I had applied earlier for Social Security disability and was receiving it since I would no longer be able to work, but the bigger issue was that of insurance. When just one of your medicines costs $12,000-$15,000 a month, and I had 2-3 more, plus Doctors' office visits, blood draws, etc, you can't go without insurance. Thankfully we were able to get COBRA, but when almost nothing is coming in, you have 2 kids in college, and with everything else life was throwing at us, this was tough. My Aunt helped us with a month and we were able to get help from the American Rescue Plan for a 2nd month. My husband looked frantically for jobs in the area, but nothing. He was able to find one 2 hours away. It would be a challenging position, but he seemed ready to take it on. This again found us living apart. Thankfully it was close enough that he could come home for weekends and other days if our youngest son had special events his senior year. We also knew it would mean another move.

Moves are hard anytime, but doubly hard when you are facing an ugly disease. So once again we started looking for a new house, and getting the one we were living in ready to sell. Packing started again, but thankfully I had gotten rid of a lot of things in the last move, so there was less stuff to pack and dispose of. The bigger problem we ended up with was that houses would come on the market and before we could even set up a visit, we would be told that the seller had accepted an offer and the house was no longer available. We finally located something that would work, was not ideal, but for now would function. We had to bid 10% over asking to get acceptance, but at least we had a place. I spent the summer prepping a 3rd house to sell.

Now the next challenge was to locate a new set of doctors. Since I have had metastatic breast cancer for 5 years now, things are only going to get more complicated and I wanted a location where I might be able to pursue clinical trials if they opened up and have an oncologist who only specialized in breast cancer. I was able to locate an excellent Oncologist at the University of Rochester, the Pluta Cancer Center. After locating a new care team, my next challenge is working to find a friend group. Never easy in the best of times, but super grateful for locating a group at the Rochester Breast Cancer Coalition.

As of the fall of 2023, my cancer has taken a turn for the worse. The cancer saw fit to find a way around Ibrance and Faslodex. It has now taken up residence in my liver also, so I am now on to a new treatment. I know the long-term outcome, but I am hoping for more time with my family, and having more time here in the Finger Lakes region. Cancer can be called the long goodbye. It tends to have one of 2 endings usually. The first is a slow extraction of things you once could do. The loss can be physical and or mental. You wonder with every celebration, holiday, or major life event, is this the last time I'll do something or see someone? The second ending is moving along losing ability and then a rapid cancer flare that fairly quickly steals what life you have left. Cancer either invades critical organs, will no longer respond to treatments, the body is so damaged it cannot take any more treatments, or creates such complications that hospice is the only recourse. Metastatic Breast Cancer is not curable, and I will be on treatment for the remainder of my life.

Even so, I am grateful for today. I am grateful for family, friends, my pets, and what I can still do, but my long-term outlook is bleak. I am living on borrowed time, and while I try to live my best, life is certainly more difficult. The bigger challenge for me now is discussing the mutations and complications from it that I may have passed on to my sons. When to get tested for the mutation and what implications it may have for their lives.

I am appreciative of what I have, but I lament what I have put my family through, and wish it could have been different. It is hard on those I love and I can't change it. Metastatic cancer has hurt me and will kill me, but I hope down the road there are more and better options for treatment, earlier detection, new medicines that are far more effective, and the ability to use in-vitro embryos that are genetically tested so this mutation is not passed on to further generations. That is my greatest solace with this cussed curse of cancer stabbing into my DNA.

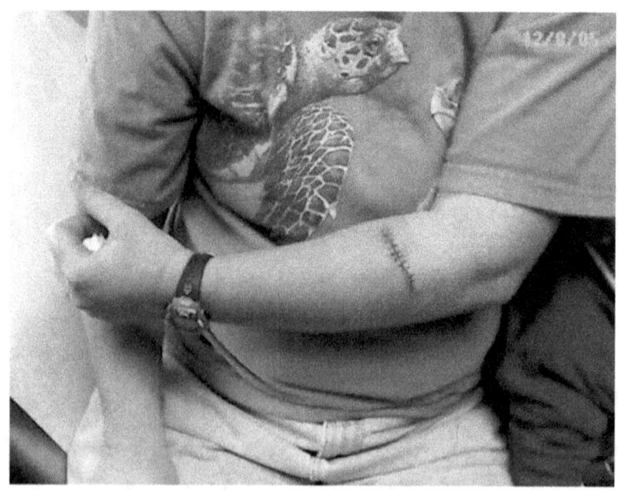

My surgery after my Melanoma

The next two stories are husband and wife.
Both had separate battles with Cancer.

12

TO WHOM MUCH IS GIVEN, MUCH WILL BE REQUIRED (LUKE 12:48)

BY ROBEN DAGHIR

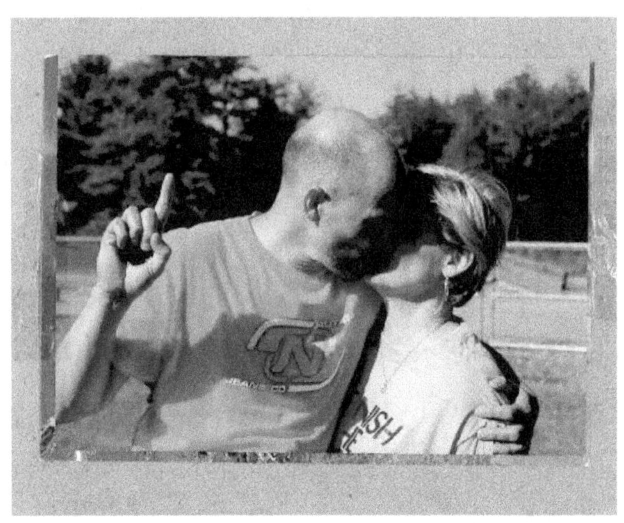

If you have heard that line of wisdom, you know it means we are held responsible for what we have. If we have been blessed with talents, wealth, knowledge, time, and the like, it is expected that we benefit others.

In 2008, I was 42 years old, happily married with twin sons (Luke & Ben) in high school and one son (Nick) in grade school. I had just completed my master's degree as a K – 12 School Counselor and was working in the high school of my hometown school district. I was healthy, happy, and content. We were enjoying the boys' activities, our family, our friendships, and looking forward to the future. Life was very busy.

In September of 2008, I had my first mammogram. It was a relatively uneventful procedure, intended to start a "baseline" for future mammograms. The day after (what should have been a "routine" mammogram), I was contacted to come in for a 2nd mammogram. The first mammogram results were "cloudy" and inconclusive. I returned the next day to the St. Marys hospital for round two. Upon conclusion of the second test, a biopsy was determined to be necessary in order to further clarify the results. I was told that the biopsy would be non-invasive and that I could return to work following the procedure. I had scheduled to be off the entire day of the biopsy despite the reassurance that returning to work was manageable. The biopsy was uncomfortable and more invasive than I had anticipated. I was reassured that 80% of breast biopsies are benign (negative). I went home to the couch following the biopsy. I recall thinking that a biopsy **is** invasive and **is** uncomfortable and stressful and anxiety filled and that the patient should **NOT** return to work the day of the procedure. A week after the biopsy, I met with Dr. J to review the pathology. He reported that the breast biopsy was malignant. He felt that a "lumpectomy" followed by chemo treatment would correct the issue. Although I felt a level of disbelief upon hearing the diagnosis, I had considered my options prior to meeting with Dr. J in the event that there was a malignancy. I told Dr. J that I wanted a mastectomy rather than a lumpectomy. I was certain that at 42 I did not want to worry about a future reoccurrence. He made arrangements for me to be seen by a surgical team in Pittsburgh 4 days later. It's amazing the details you remember and the things you forget as you learn of a cancer diagnosis. Dr. J hugged me before I left his office. I remember thinking the hug from Dr. J was shocking but kind. I was not prepared for his hug. I recall feeling awkward that he had his arms around my "unlifted" arms that were down at my side. I recall having an "Ally McBeal" moment where I realized he was genuinely concerned for me. Although he was reassuring me….it wasn't. He instructed me to go to Paulette Schreiber's office (Women's Care) down the hall upon leaving him. Paulette was aware of my diagnosis and was prepared to consult with me before sending me out on my own. I went home and casually told my husband that the test results said breast cancer. His reply was, "really…go tell the boys". The twins were in the basement goofing around. I told them that I have breast cancer. They stopped what they were doing, looked up in shock, paused quietly for a moment and then replied, "It's going to be ok". I replied, "yes, it will". I then went next door to my parents' home to deliver the news of my newly identified breast cancer. From there I notified my siblings, neighbors, friends, and eventually coworkers. Some people had been aware that I was having a biopsy. Due to numerous reasons…. the news spread throughout my world like rocket fire. I was immediately met with compassion. My age may have contributed to the sharing of my diagnosis. Many of the students in the high school could identify with concern as I was close in age with their mothers. Students shared their concern with my high school sons. Nicholas stood up on the bus and told the other riders, "My mom has cancer right here" as he touched his shirt. I was overwhelmed by the shift in the culture at work. I felt supported by staff and students. What could have been a lonely and frightening event was ultimately a positive experience." I was faced with an undesired scenario. At no point do I recall feeling alone on the journey. I felt empowered by the love and support we received. I would only later find out that while I was in the hospital and throughout my recovery, many of my students reached out to my sons seeking updates and lending their support. I felt grateful for the life I have and the communities to which I belong.

Off to Pittsburgh for the next leg of the race. I was notified in our first appointment in Pittsburgh that I had "strings of cancerous cells that filled most of the right breast. I did not yet have a "lump" that could have been detected in a self-exam. My options were never a lumpectomy and treatment. I had to choose between the loss of ½ or the entire right breast. Very few things made me nauseous or queasy. The thought of losing ½ the breast was something I found to be repulsive. Due to my overall good health and relatively young age, I was given the option of a bilateral mastectomy with reconstruction. I was informed that "I had time to make a decision… but I should hurry up". I was offered a bilateral mastectomy with trans flap. Due to my having "extra" reserve stomach fat from my pregnancies, I was offered a tummy tuck. My abdomen fat would be rolled up under the skin to form new breasts. It didn't take much discerning and we had decided to have the bilateral surgery with recon-struction. I was told it would be a hard hit up front with the rewards to follow thereafter. I would initially feel like I "was hit by a Mack truck" but removal of all of the breast tissue would lower the risk of a future reoccurrence. Looking back, everything in Pittsburgh was gracefully unfolding. The surgeons, plastic surgeons, technicians, and hospital personnel were very conscious of our lengthy drive for treatment. Most of our appointments and procedures were scheduled back-to-back to accommodate our travel. We scheduled the 12-hour bilateral mastectomy for October 31, 2008 (Halloween).

On October 30th, Joe, my parents, and I trekked off to Pitts-burgh to stay the night before the very early surgery. I remember feeling motivated, grateful, and loved. I remember feeling that I just wanted to get it all over with and put it behind us. I was eager to move forward and return to my "new" normal. Being the patient is the easy part. Joe and my parents waited and paced for the entire day until the surgery was complete. I have very little recollection of the course of events. I woke up in my room where I would stay for the week. I recall waking up feeling extremely nauseous, confused, exhausted and uncomfortable. I woke up to my sister and her husband at my bedside with Joe. My parents were nearby. Our boys were safely supervised with my twin brother Bob and his wife Kelly in St. Marys. I was extremely comfortable with the boys' arrangements. I genuinely didn't give them a second thought. It didn't take long for me to realize that "it takes a village", we truly are **all** in this together, and I have to get better before I can even consider taking care of my family again. My brother and sister-in-law brought our boys to Pittsburgh once during the week to help them understand the gravity of the circumstances. When people offer to help out, they mean it. It doesn't make us weak to accept support (financial, babysitting, cleaning, shopping, mowing the lawn). If people offer to help-don't hesitate to take them up on it. People need and want to feel useful.

Returning home brought on a whole new kind of exhaustion. I went home from the hospital with "drainage" tubes. One drainage tube coming from each "new" breast and one from each side of my abdomen. I had 4 drainage tubes in total. Initially, I felt as though the "discharge" was disgusting and vial. Joe didn't hesitate to assist in my daily regimen of care. He emptied and reattached those bulbs on the end of the drainage tubes without even wincing. I recall having very strong senses. I was repulsed by "myself". There was vial liquid draining from my body. My stitches "smelled" of dried blood. The smell of "hand sanitizer" was offensive. While in the hospital, prior to any interaction from medical staff, they would amply sanitize their hands with sanitizer. Immediately thereafter, health professionals would adjust the tubes around my nose which sent the sanitizer scent up through my olfactory bulb making the scent an ongoing negative reminder of the trauma of the hospital setting. The strong alcohol scent can still negatively trigger me to this day.

I came home to the support of a community nurse. Her name is Jackie. She grew up in my neighborhood and I've known her my whole life. She is a phenomenal nurse and even more amazing person. She was direct and very real. I relayed to her that I felt like I wanted to "thrash" my head left and right often and couldn't adjust to a comfortable sitting or lying position. Jackie informed me that that feeling is called "pain". Taking my prescriptions as directed became a very important aspect of the recovery. The trick was to stay "ahead" of the pain. Over time, every day the pain was a little less intense. My appetite eventually returned. I remember having the 'ability" to lay down and sleep anywhere/anytime. Sometimes I **wanted** to lay down, other times I **had** to lay down. Recovery from any surgery, illness, or accident requires patience. We were blessed to received daily dinners from friends, neighbors, family, and coworkers. Our community blessed us daily with cards, gifts, money, phone calls, and prayers. The mailbox was full of cards and there were gifts and treats on our front porch for weeks. The outreach was amazing and often too much to comprehend. I often wondered why we received so much support when I don't recall ever being that generous with others … ever. Again, there were moments of fear and frustration but never a moment of loneliness. People had our backs. I saved many of the cards and emails I received throughout the diagnosis and recovery. One of my favorites cards was from our neighbor Adam. He put the card on our windshield the night before we left for the surgery in Pittsburgh. We found it in the morning and still laugh. The card went something like this, "Don't worry, my aunt had this surgery and now she's my uncle". The humor really was that I was going in for a life changing female surgery/alteration. The card hit home and was humbling at the same time. Very clever. My greatest obstacle in recovery was the abdominal pain I felt from the trans flap/tummy tuck procedure. I was cut from hip to hip. The pain was something I had never before experienced, even from my c-section deliveries. I returned to work after 10 weeks of recovery. It was upon my "return" to "normal" life that I realized my role had changed.

I was eager to return to my high school position. I missed my coworkers and the students….and the routine. I needed a schedule and a purpose. Again, I was overwhelmed by the support I received. I had the opportunity to speak at a school wide assembly about my experience. I was met with resounding support from the high school community. My close coworker, Jeff, who has a solid comedic side surprised me one day with his observations. He told me, "You are different" to which I replied, "I know". He said, "No… you aren't afraid anymore". I genuinely was moved by his statement and realized there was truth behind it. Yes, yes, I had changed. And yes, yes, I wasn't afraid anymore. The diagnosis and surgery and recovery and relief and support and ability to return to my former self…. all had made me stronger and just different. I felt a compelling clarity and reality that life is a gift. We aren't guaranteed the rest of today much less tomorrow. I realized that I cared more about some things and not a whole lot about other things. I felt an inner strength and appreciation for the gifts I have been given. I felt a desire to make my mark on this earth and possibly help someone else, somehow, some way. I felt a strong desire to continue to learn and share and support the people around me and people I haven't yet met. I felt a strong spiritual connection to my faith and a close relationship with Jesus Christ. I experienced other feelings that were new to me. As I became a "poster child" for women experiencing a breast cancer diagnosis, I began to feel remorse and shame and guilt that I was a survivor when so many others did not survive. I felt appreciation for the women who went through cancer before me. The women who did not win their cancer battle. The women who fought for their lives and tried new treatments and trials. Those treatments eventually were perfected and saved my life. I will always be appreciative to those women. They remind me to work hard to get to Heaven so that I can meet them and thank them one day. Ultimately, there were roller coaster days of highs and lows for a very long time. I felt rejuvenated more than I felt ever before. Until…

13

MY CANCER STORY

BY JOE DAGHIR

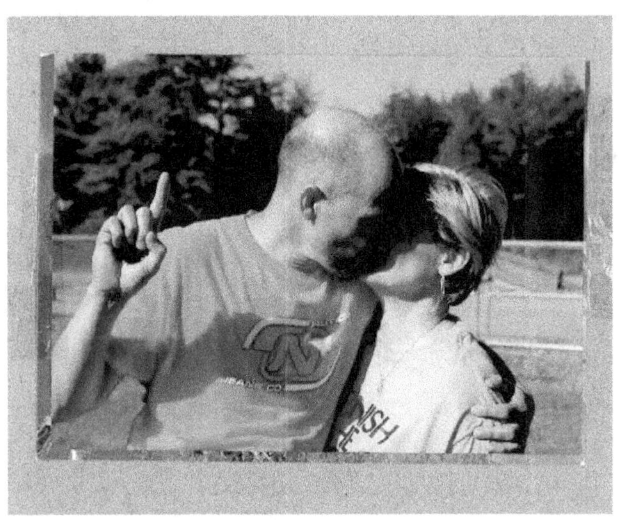

In 2007, one of my older siblings was diagnosed with Colorectal cancer. Medical protocol recommends that siblings undergo a colonoscopy when a sibling is diagnosed.

My first "scope" was performed at Elk Regional Hospital in 2007. The doctor reported, "All Good" following the procedure. He instructed me to seek another colonoscopy in 5 years, 2012. I accepted my results and went on with my life. I experienced no concerns throughout 2008. In 2009, my stools began to change from solid to soft/loose. This continued into 2010. I spoke with my doctor. He appeared to have little concern. I began to experience shooting pains in my groin area while driving throughout 2011. In 2012, blood periodically appeared in my bowel movements. (Listen to your body!!) I told my wife, Roben, about my symptoms and by the look on her face, I knew she was concerned.

We went through cancer with Roben in 2008 (at the actual time my cancer likely began). I never thought we would get on this train again. I was 47 years old at this time. I scheduled my second colonoscopy with Dr. F. at the Elk Regional Hospital for 02/12/2012. Dr. F. is a wonderful doctor working with a wonderful team. Her nurse Melissa was very helpful. A tumor was found in the 2nd scope. The tumor was the size of a golf ball and located in my rectum. A tissue sample was taken. The lab report confirmed cancer. The cancer was identified as invasive adenocarcinoma of the colon.

Dr. F. immediately made our referral to an oncology surgeon affiliated with UPMC Pittsburgh. Dr. F. relayed that "This cancer needs removed and depending upon staging, possibly chemo." Not what Roben and I wanted to hear. Our life was good, why this, God? We had young kids! We had already gone through this with Roben, why now, God!! During the 5-minute ride home after learning my diagnosis, not a word was spoken between us. No sooner had we walked into the house when two of my coworkers showed up with balloons and jokes about the colonoscopy! FUNNY! A rather awkward visit. We did not tell them the truth of the findings at that time. We took a drive to camp to walk our dogs. This was the same walk we took when Roben was diagnosed in 2008. This walk would give us time alone to begin to process what the hell had just happened! As we walked and began to talk a beautiful snowfall began. We were at peace. Dr. F. called us again that same night. She had consulted with our family doctor. They had scheduled a PET scan with fusion at Clarion Hospital mobile scan unit on 02/28/12. I asked why this was needed. Dr F. said this would confirm if the cancer had broken through the colon and metastasized to other areas in my body. Once again, Roben and I were terrified. Dr. F. sensed our fear and told us to come to her office. What a beautiful lady. She took the time to listen and she informed us of what she thought was on the horizon.

The 16 days we waited for the PET scan were tough. On 02/28/12, I drove to Clarion Hospital mobile scan and arrived at 8AM. A tech handed me a "robe" with instructions and a brief chat about the procedure. All I can say is that this scan stuff was a cold place, and I began to experience fear; lots of fear! Bad thoughts began to flood my head. I stopped the bad thoughts and fear with prayer. I asked Jesus to take care of my family. As simple as that …I felt comfort! Fear and anxiety would be a thorn in my ass for the next year. Prayer would get me through the bad times. After the scan, the tech opened the door and tossed my bagged clothes on the slab. "Get dressed, see you, your doctor will call you". That's it! No hug! I chuckled as I walked by the dude and out the mobile unit. The waiting period for the scan results was tough on Roben. We did not tell family yet. We wanted to know the facts before we confided with loved ones.

Two days after the scan, my family doctor called with great news. "The cancer is contained to the groin area and did not metastasize." The best words ever heard! Dr C. and Dr. F called me daily. Later on, family and friends called often as well. The calls from family and friends were big medicine.

Both doctors confirmed that surgery must happen sooner than later.

Now it was time to tell the kids. We knew I would make it. Telling little Nick was easy, he was 10. He needed reassurance that his life would not change drastically. Telling the twins was tough; they came home from college over the weekend. They were loving life and not expecting to hear dad has cancer! Comments from them, "will you make it? We hear chemo is tough". Roben worked her magic and we got that behind us. In her loving way she assured the kids we all will be ok. That talk set the tone!! It was good to tell family and friends. I was relieved that we were no longer alone.

A side note – crazy…for some reason I began to work out daily in 2011. I got myself in the best physical shape ever. Was this God's plan? It prepared me for the tough fight ahead.

Roben and I talked more than ever. Family and friends began to shower us with cards, food, calls, visits and money. We were stunned with the love we received from the community. Not just our parish at St. Mary's, but all of Elk County seemed to step up.

An ultrasound was scheduled for March 8th, 2012, at Presbyterian Hospital in Pittsburgh. This procedure, called Endo sonographic rectal ultrasound, was performed by Dr. Jen C. This procedure positively identified the location of the tumor as well as the involved malignant lymph nodes. My cancer was staged at uT3 un1 with sonographic evidence of invasion into the 5th layer of the muscularis propria and no evidence of metastasizes. I later found out that the above means that I had stage 3 cancer and surgery was required ASAP.

Roben and I were given the names of four surgeons at UMPC. We went with Dr. C.'s preferred surgeon, Dr. G. Dr. G called me on my cell phone late one night and was the only surgeon to call me. He said he could remove the cancer by surgery and I would not have a colonoscopy bag.

Dr. G and his team reviewed all the tests and scans and scheduled surgery March 27th, 2012, at St. Margaret's

Hospital. I was so relieved; I was finally getting this cancer out of me! March 24th, 2012, Dr G's office called and bumped up surgery to March 26th, 2012. I was ordered to use another colon cleanse (I would do a thousand of them before having cancer surgery, radiation and chemo).

Our youngest son Nick was getting his Arrow of Light award from the boy scouts on March 25th. Unfortunately, I missed it due to my surgery. I am very proud of my 3 boys all earning their Eagle Award. Thankfully, Bob and Aunt Kelly stepped up again and took care of Nick, so Roben and I never had to worry about him. Thanks Bob and Kelly! They took Nick to his Arrow of Light award and supported him at that moment. Roben and I are so blessed with family and friends. Thank you all.

Roben and I booked a room near St. Margaret's and prepared for the surgery scheduled for March 26th. We were exhausted. We missed the kids and our family. I was relieved when we got to the hospital at 5AM, as directed. My job was done. Now it was up to the surgical team. As I reflect on that time, I can't thank family enough, for reducing my stress by taking care of everything else.

March 27, 2012, I remember a nurse talking with Roben with concern that I was so weak. Dr. G. visited my room and told Roben that I had lost a lot of blood and needed a blood transfusion. I got the blood. Thanks to whoever donated! I was in the hospital for 9 days. We celebrated my birthday in Room 525. Great party! I love you Roben. Thanks for staying in room 525, sleeping on the cot, and being the gate keeper to keep family and all visitors out! I did not want illness/viruses coming in and it worked.

The twins came for a visit and realized how weak I was. Shock was the expression on their face. I felt bad putting them in the middle of this. They stepped up and helped with my recovery for the next year. After 9 days, I was excited to get my walking papers and I got the hell out of St. Margaret's. The ride home was agonizing. Every bump rattled my body with pain. I thought to myself, "How can I do this at home? I can't even sit up, let alone walk"! The surgery required my abdomen to be cut from 5 inches below my midline to one inch below my belly button. Roben and our neighbor bought a recliner for me to recover in. Best thing having the recliner!! I could not get up from the couch or chair because my core was cut open. No strength and I had to learn to roll out of the recliner and bed! Again, surgery by far was the hardest on me. My brother Chop and his family took care of our very active young puppy.

Some recollections from that time are positive. I remember pulling in the driveway after the release from the hospital. Family and friends placed signs, "WELCOME home JOE", along the driveway. It was good to be home. It was also very hard to be home. I only had enough strength to walk 100 feet on the sidewalk! Roben made sure I did the walk 3 times per day. In a month I could "shuffle" around the block.

I weighed 184 pounds pre surgery and in May I weighed 140lbs. I began my treatment at Hahne Cancer Center in DuBois with Dr. M. His team was wonderful. He told Roben and I that I would do well with the chemo treatments. He ordered a chemo port along with a portable chemo pump. The chemo port was another surgery. I was told that this was not a big deal and it was scheduled in one week. I got the port in and got C-DIF! Not a good thing to get when one is weak. C-DIF is a nasty intestinal illness that kills. I began to have uncontrolled diarrhea along with my stomach rolling and shifting from the stress the intestines had endured. Luckily Dr. G's nurse called in a medication for me immediately. I started the medication the same day I became ill. This nurse's immediate action cleared up the C-DIF in 2 days.

I met with Dr. M. and his team, and I met all the staff and was given a tour of the infusion room. The room was painted to make you feel relaxed but I knew this was a tough place to be. I later realized that I was wrong about this place. This room was going to save me and bond me with fellow survivors. This room changed me for the better. This room got the cancer out of me.

Dr M. developed a cocktail of drugs best suited for me (included Fluoracil Solution, 5 FU, Oxaliplatin along with Leucovarin). The cocktail went along with 32 radiation treatments. I was not happy about the news of radiation. I fought this until Roben got me back on track. I was mad at the world and tired of subjecting myself to everything. Little did I know that radiation was not so bad on me. I felt bad after I saw the women with burn marks who were fighting breast cancer. I got to know them in the brief 10-minute radiation treatment. I only got radiation for approximately 30 seconds! That was it, then I was out the door.

I wanted my old life back, happy go lucky Joe. I had to keep remembering how lucky I was. Blessed may be the best word! I began my recovery when I bought into the chemo and radiation team. Dr. K., Radiation Oncologist, is a wonderful soft-spoken gentleman. I was not going to get radiation by my choice but Roben again took charge and set me in my place (Thanks Honey).

I began to receive small amounts of the chemo cocktail via the portable pump along with radiation. According to the doctor, this combo of treatment enhanced recovery. I had a coworker friend stop by one night and he had suffered a life changing illness years back. Dinner with Jim was my turning point to recovery; thanks for stopping.

I realized how blessed I was to be a Hahne patient. I met beautiful people and many cancer survivors. They gave me strength and hope. I lost two great friends during the nine months of treatment, great people who sat next to me in the chemo chairs biweekly; Mark and Bill. God called them home. Those two guys were my rock! I began to suffer from survivor guilt, why them and not me? Losing them was tough. Looking at the empty chemo chairs they normally sat in was tough. The staff at Hahne knew what I was going through. They were so compassionate and comforted us as we struggled. Thank you all! Thank you, Steph, for the powerful words you told me "Are you going to be a big boy and drive yourself to treatment next time?" Well, I did and I began to live. I learned to get through the survivor guilt by living every day for my fellow patients! I began to see the simple things in life and appreciate what matters. I began to look into people's eyes when we talked. I began to become a better person. Thank you Hahne, you know me and I know you. Along with other survivors; we love you!

Roben gave me a book written by Lance Armstrong about his story with cancer. Lance kept his port after it was removed from his chest…so did Joe Daghir. This man-made instrument reminds me of what I was and what I must be. I hold this port in my hand as a reminder of the tough time and as a reminder to live!

God got me through the year of treatment and recovery. God and family, friends and a pigeon named George! Nick and Ry girl remember George the pigeon. Thank you, neighbors (The Hood)!! It was a rough ride but you all made it doable.

Nick, remember chemo buck? Your first buck in German settlement the same day of my last treatment! Thanks for pushing me to live!

To all thank you! My recovery was because of you! Thanks Elk County Relay for Life! Thanks, Roben, Love you!

14

SHOCK OF A LIFETIME

BY SARA SHREFLER

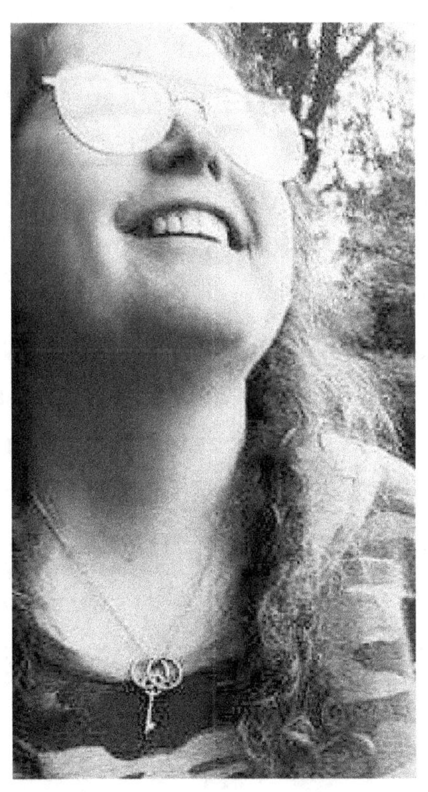

I found out I had a brain tumor in 2011, but it was long before then that I felt the symptoms. It was around 2007 when it first started. At first it was just forgetting little things, like going to the laundromat and forgetting the detergent, but this memory problem caused me to lose my job. I was forgetting to do certain things and it was affecting my judgement terribly. Following an incredibly careless choice, I got fired from my job. Next came the severe headaches. They were so bad they would make me vomit. I thought I was going crazy; I was seeing things that weren't there. My family was also very concerned, so I had my mom take me to DuBois hospital so I could commit myself to the psych ward. It was not helping. I got on antidepressants and anti-anxiety meds, but they didn't help either. It got so bad that I stopped caring about my appearance. I let my home fall into disarray. Normally I was OCD about myself and my home being clean, but I was in too much pain to care. My father thought I was into drugs because of the company I was keeping; he would later come to regret saying that to me. Then the seizures began. I knew when they were coming. I would kind of black out only for a second or two, but then I would hear this buzzing sound in my head. Next thing I knew I would be on the ground, wondering how I got there, while being unable to get up. Of course, I addressed my issues with my family doctor, and she dismissed the headaches as a sinus infection. I was given so many antibiotics between 2007-2011, but nothing would help this "sinus infection" go away. The last seizure was the worst one I experienced. I fell down about 30 steps outside of my home and hit my head on the road at the bottom of the steps. At that time, I was working for a home health care company and living with a less than stellar boyfriend, but I wouldn't realize just how "not stellar" he was until after my brain surgery. He would drop me off in the mornings at my job and pick me up when it was time to go home. But after I fell down the steps, I needed him to step up. I told him he needed to take me to the ER because I had a seizure and fell down the outside steps. He was griping about it, saying he had "plans" that day, but eventually he took me. My boyfriend just dropped me off at the hospital door and told me to call him when I was ready to come home, but that call never came.

After I told the ER doctor what happened, they wheeled me to get a CT scan. I think I must have blacked out, because next thing I remember was a nurse telling me that I couldn't be treated at that hospital. Because they found a mass in my brain, she asked me where I would like to be treated, Pittsburgh or Erie. I chose Pittsburgh, since my father had experienced several benign brain tumors and that's where he was treated. I was life flighted to UPMC Presby. I remember waking up on the roof of the hospital and this lady from the helicopter was trying to put a brace on my neck, and I was fighting her telling her I didn't want it.

Next thing I remember was waking up in a recovery room surrounded by my family, and asking them what happened. They told me I had a craniotomy where they removed a large lemon sized tumor from my brain, which they had to biopsy to determine if it was cancerous. Indeed, it was. I was so shocked but actually kind of relived that I wasn't crazy. Now I knew what was causing my awful headaches, not a sinus infection, just a cancerous brain tumor. The surgeon informed me that when he made the cut into my skull, the tumor just started to pop out. That's how much pressure was inside my head. He also told me that he couldn't remove all of it, because if he did, he would run the risk of giving me permanent brain damage, but that I was lucky to be alive. My tumor was an anaplastic astrocytoma, which is very slow growing, which explains a lot of my symptoms. It was then that my cell phone rang; it was my boyfriend looking to see if I was ready to be picked up yet. My mom answered it and said "No asshole, she's been life flighted to Pittsburgh, and I'm going to need you to get your stuff out of her house and return her keys to her cousin, because she's going to be here for a while. She had a cancerous brain tumor, and when she is released from the hospital, she's going to be living with me and my sister and brother-in-law in Harrisburg." I had no say in this decision, since I couldn't really function on my own and I knew my boyfriend was not up to the task.

I was in Presby NICU (Neurology Intensive Care Unit) for several weeks. I was not accepting my diagnosis yet. I had a

Billy Bag on the back of my head to drain the blood and discharge from my surgery, and a catheter since I couldn't walk. I got lucky because my nurse was a Steelers fan, so he put on the games for me. My mom slept in the waiting room the entire time I was in the NICU. I would doze in and out of sleep, because they had me on a morphine drip. Every time I woke up, I asked for my mom. Her youngest sister was there too, but my dad couldn't stay. The day I was diagnosed with brain cancer, his wife had told him that she had breast cancer and had known for several months, but she was Japanese, and thought she could cure herself without chemotherapy or a mastectomy. She passed away a few years later, after she decided to try chemo. But by then it was too late, her cancer spread to her lungs and eventually her bones…she was just a shell by the time she passed.

Eventually they removed my catheter and my drainage bag and I was moved to a private room, but I still had to ring for the nurse every time I needed to go to the bathroom. Since I had been in a bed immobilized for several weeks, my legs became weak and I couldn't walk without assistance. It was in this private room that I finally accepted my diagnosis. I had one little boo-hoo moment where I cried, and then decided that this cancer would not kill me. It was decided that I would be treated at Penn State Hershey Cancer Institute.

When I was finally released from the hospital, I had a great support system in Harrisburg. I was living with my Aunt

Jean and Uncle Lou and their kitties. I was set up in the fully finished basement, and my aunt worked from home so she took care of me when my mom was at work. I also had a good support system back in Elk County, where friends and family held benefits for me to assist in my precarious financial situation. I was obviously unable to work or drive for about a year, and this year was no vacation. Since I was set up in the basement, I was unable to climb the stairs fast enough to make it to the bathroom on time, so my aunt provided me with a handicapped toilet. My brain was unable to process when I had to go, so I had to wear adult diapers for quite some time. I eventually got all my belongings out of my house and kept my Jeep at my dad's until I could drive again. This is when I learned that the man I had been living with was selling drugs out of my Jeep. My dad found a stolen checkbook and a bottle of Ritalin in someone else's name in my Jeep. I was horrified. I had to let the bank take my house because I could no longer pay my mortgage. I had to file for bankruptcy, but I was able to keep my Jeep, since the money raised from the benefits and fundraisers was enough to make the payments on my Jeep. I had 5 cats and my cousin fed them until I was able to get them to Harrisburg. My Aunt Jean and Uncle Lou were cat lovers so they didn't mind, as long as I kept their litter boxes clean. For this I am eternally grateful, because they were my emotional support at that time.

Eventually we got a U-Haul and completed getting my belongings out of my house. I couldn't bring my queen-sized bed to my aunt's house, but I had a daybed, which my aunt kindly set up in her craft room, which was on the first floor of her home. The rest of my stuff went into storage. We had to live by my aunt and uncle's rules, which meant church every Sunday, which was not fun. But I met a lot of great people at their church, and it got me out of the house.

Before undergoing treatment at Hershey Med, I had to go back to Presby for a follow-up on my surgery. It was there that I was told my prognosis wasn't good, but my dad drilled into my head daily positive thought only. I had no idea what to expect for my treatment, so I was set up with a neuro-oncologist, who was awesome, and actually listened to me; I was put on many scripts, including Keppra, which is an anti-seizure medication that I have to be on for the rest of my life, and steroids to help with inflammation. The steroids made me eat like a bloodthirsty pig and caused me to gain quite a bit of weight, and as an added bonus, they gave me terrible acne and a moon face. I had several rounds of radiation, for which I had to be fitted with a mask before I had the moon face, so it fit when they made it, but once I started the radiation during my "moon face" stage, it squeezed my head painfully. I had to have radiation at least 2x per week, which left me exhausted. Simply put, my radiation oncologist was kind of a non-supportive jerk. He left to go somewhere with his family for Thanksgiving and bluntly told me he didn't expect to see me when he returned. I proved him wrong. While receiving radiation, I was also taking a chemo pill called Temodar, which made me violently ill and caused my hair to start falling out. The day I woke up and saw my hair all over my pillow, I requested my aunt to shave it off. I cried while she did this, although my surgeon had already given me a super cool haircut, insert sarcasm. It was a reverse Mohawk. I had 57 staples in my head shaped kind of like a horseshoe, and one of them got infected, so now I have a permanent dent in my head, and the right side of my hair is pretty sparse, since that's where all scar tissue sits. I opted to typically wear hats instead of wigs, but I often wore a pink wig I got from the Halloween rack at Walmart, because I was a punk rocker. My hair grew back slowly, but it came back a lighter shade of brown and curly. I wasn't mad. At least I didn't need my curling iron anymore.

When I was done with radiation, I moved on to infusions of chemotherapy. My poison was called Avastin, it was not a cure, it just prevented what was left of my tumor from growing. At first it was like twice a week, then once a week, then every two weeks, until it was once every three months. It didn't make me sick, but I couldn't function the day after an infusion. It just zapped my energy. My neuro oncologist finally took me off the steroids, and my face was starting to look normal again. I lost about 100lbs very rapidly, so now I am full of stretch marks, which I wear proudly, for they are my battle scars.

Now, almost 13 years later I am not receiving Avastin anymore, but my neuro oncologist wants me to get MRIs every three months instead of every four, which I am fine with. I am grateful that I no longer have to mainline poison anymore. I will never be the same again, I struggle with many things that most people take for granted. I get dizzy a lot, I struggle with stairs, I still have problems controlling my bladder and bowels, I have to sit down to get dressed or I will fall over. I have to sit down to put my shoes on, I struggle at making decisions, and my memory kind of sucks now, but throughout all of these issues, I am so very grateful and truly blessed to be alive. As of October of 2023, my MRIs haven't changed. And as of March of 2023, I haven't received Avastin.

One thing that really helped me was staying positive. So I say to you the reader: if you are faced with a life-altering diagnosis, always stay positive and never take the time you have for granted.

THE SERENITY PRAYER

> *God Grant me the Serenity to accept the things I*
> *cannot change*
> *The Courage to change the things I can*
> *And The Wisdom to know the difference*

MY TUMOR, THEY REMOVED

Before

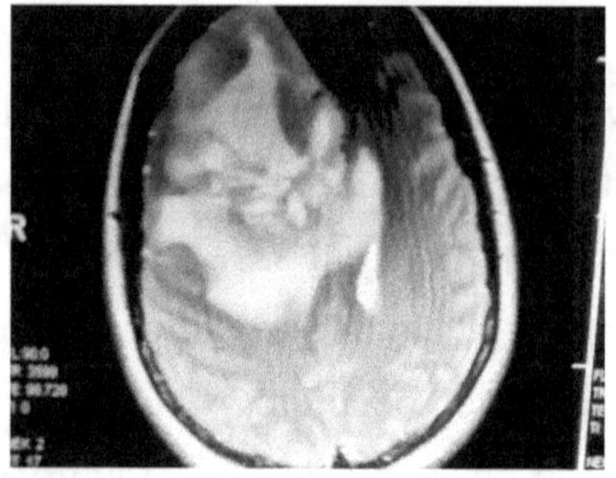

After

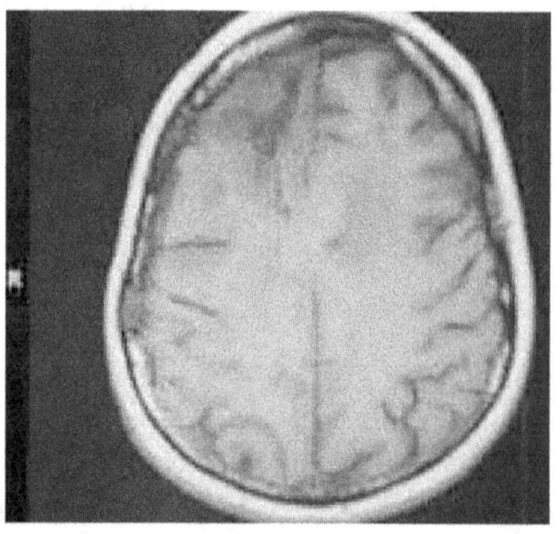

15

THE UPS AND DOWNS OF RECOVERY,

MY JOURNEY THROUGH CANCER

BY TINA ORNER

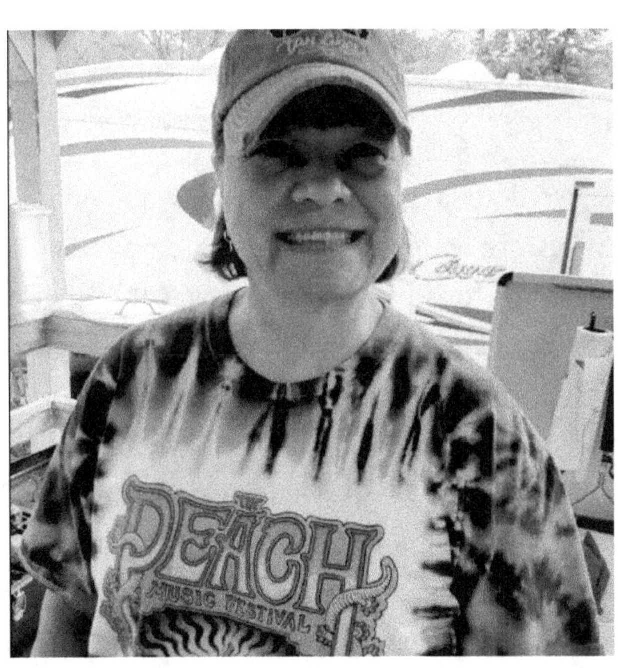

My journey started in 2001. In February, I helped my boyfriend recover from a heart-attack. In March, I had to have my gall bladder removed. In April, I found a lump in my right breast. My general practitioner sent me for a mammogram where the lump was confirmed, resulting in having an ultrasound. I had bought a book titled *"Dr. Susan Love's Breast Book"* and I read it cover to cover. I found out that if during the ultrasound the lump looks smooth and wavy it is most likely is not cancerous. But, if the lump looks like it has finger-like jagged edges, it might be cancer reaching out to the rest of your body. I remember the technician telling me that she had to speak to the doctor, and as she left I peeked over at the screen, and I saw the finger-looking edges of the lump. I knew then that it was not going to be a good outcome.

I was referred to a general surgeon who did the needle biopsy in his office. It was only a few days later that I was called to the doctor's office where I was told that although the biopsy showed no cancer, the surgeon said he would like to do a lumpectomy because he did not like the outcome of the ultrasound. This doctor probably saved my life! I believe that had he not gone this avenue, the cancer could have spread and the outcome would not have been the same. I will never forget the phone call from the surgeon telling me that the tumor was indeed cancer. I think he was just as upset as I was. Since the cancer was positive he offered me two options – one was to go back in and take more tissue from around where the lump was (lumpectomy) or have a mastectomy. I chose the latter.

When my boyfriend came home from work, I was standing next to my dresser in my bedroom. I told him the doctor had called and my biopsy was positive for cancer. He never left my side all through my treatment and everything else I had to go through. He was there to support me. I have heard from other women that their husbands/boyfriends left them because of the mastectomies and treatments. I was very fortunate to have him by my side.

My niece was a nurse who worked in local hospital administration. She knew the best doctors in all the fields in my area. She is the one that gave me the names of the general surgeon, plastic surgeon, and oncology doctors who I wound up using.

Next came the surgery for my mastectomy, along with the placement of an expander under the muscle in my breast to stretch the muscle and skin to make room for a permanent implant. My surgeon called me the night before my surgery to check on me. He really helped me feel safe, going into such an experience.

I started the chemotherapy and injections in the expander pretty quickly after my surgery. Zofran was my friend to control the nausea from my treatment. It was a rough six months between the weekly chemo treatments and twice a week injections to fill my expander, followed by the reconstruction surgery and recovery. I did a lot of needlepoint during the chemo treatments.

During all these months, I worked my full-time job as an electronic mechanic at our local army depot and as a part time head cashier at Home Depot. I was lucky that both jobs allowed me to work around my busy schedule of doctors' visits and chemo treatments and for those days that I was not up to going to work. The team of co-workers at both places were so accommodation and compassionate that it made life so much easier for me.

One of the things I missed most during my treatment and recovery was riding our motorcycle. We took a break so I could get back to feeling comfortable on the bike, and then I began riding again. Although I had a wig, I mostly wore baseball caps or Harley Doo-rags. I felt like a real badass chick being bald from the chemo and all leathered up!

I volunteered for many groups during my treatment. I was interviewed for a newspaper article and television spots. I just wanted to get the word out that there is help, you just have to ask for it. I manned tables at different events, and I would do different speaking engagements discussing options for those recently diagnosed. I would talk about simple things like, wearing a man's tee-shirt under your mastectomy bra after surgery for more comfort, and seeking out special robes that could hold the drain tubes and bulbs after surgery. I also tell those recently diagnosed to listen to what the doctors and nurses tell you to do, they are trained professionals and deal with helping patients every day. Another piece of advice is to rest when you need to; don't worry about the dishes, the laundry or any other housework, it will get done sometime. Don't hesitate to ask for help, this is a hard thing to do for most women. People that say "Let me know if you need anything" CALL them, take them up on their offer! Remember you are not alone in this journey.

I was fortunate to have my son, siblings, and other family members readily available to help me through those tough and trying years.

I made so many friends that also volunteered with me and we have become lifelong friends. We have had many ups and downs, but always we know we are only a phone call away. I cherish our many outings, even if it is just a cup of coffee and a donut. Some of get together at times and go out for a nice dinner.

While I was looking for a wig to wear since I knew my hair was going to fall out from the chemo, I found a shop called "That Special Woman". While I was there, I was told about a new camp called "Camp Bravehearts," an oncology camp for women. This camp was pretty new and just becoming established. My boyfriend was with me and quickly pulled the camp fee out of his pocket and said, "You need to sign up!" He thought it was a great organization, so I signed up! He was so right! With that membership, I entered a group of wonderful women all on a fabulous trek through time and recovery. I was able to participate with meeting groups of ladies that all had something in common: Cancer! I was hooked. I showed up after the chemo treatments, bald with a Harley ball cap on, wearing a t-shirt with Betty Boop sitting on a Harley Davidson Motorcycle. I also had my jeans and Harley boots on. Some of the gals were a little intimated about this "Biker Chick" but quickly we because the best of friends. So, right from the start my nickname was Betty Boop or just Boop.

After a few years, I was asked to become a member of the all-volunteer staff, which was a position I quickly accepted. I have been in charge of ordering merchandise and selling it at our camp retreats as a means of making money to keep the camp going. It continues to be a comfortable group effort, as we all have similar ideas and we work well together.

Since my diagnosis, I have retired from federal service after almost 38 years on the job. Along with working part time for Home Depot during those years, I spent several years at Macy's after leaving the government, having some interesting moments and enjoying working retail. Later, I worked fulfilling online orders for a Grammy winning artist. That was pretty cool. These days, I am really just enjoying retirement. Bravehearts keeps me busy as well, and I have been helping family members that are recovering from illnesses.

Life has not been easy though. In the past five years alone, I have lost my mom and my twin sister, had a reoccurrence resulting in a second mastectomy, survived a stroke and had several surgeries. I also survived two bouts of Covid!

In 2022, I was blessed with welcoming my daughter-in-law, Sameen, into my family. My son Bill and Sameen make my life very happy. Whatever I need, they are right there for me. Even a ton of their friends treat me like their own mother and friend. My life is complete.

I do not know what the future has in store for me, but I know I will not be alone.

16

BEST FRIENDS FOR LIFE
BY MARY ANNE MEEKER

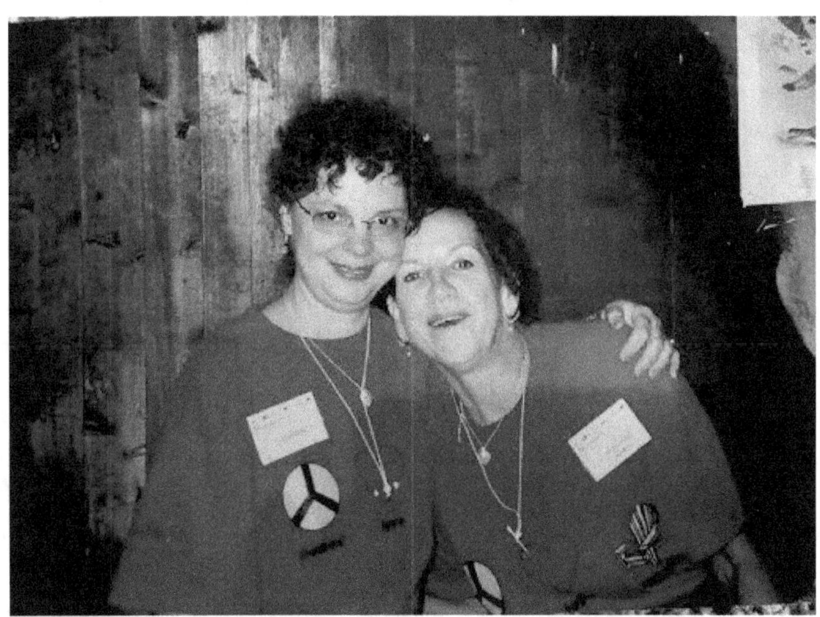

In February 1996, I went for my annual gyno check which included a breast exam. Prior to this visit I had a mammogram in October 1995, which was negative. The doctor noticed something suspicious and immediately sent me for a breast ultrasound. While at work (as a nurse in a physician's office), the doctor called me and said the results of the ultrasound warranted a further look and referred me to a surgeon. The surgeon referred me to the American Cancer Society's Reach to Recovery Program where I met Carol Marino, who turned out to be a life-long friend. She visited me at my home prior to my surgery. She told me her story and I was impressed about the fact that she had a tram-flap reconstruction following her mastectomy. I did some research and thought it might be a good idea for me to look into this for myself. As it turned out I was a good candidate for this procedure and I was scheduled for a mastectomy and tram-flap reconstruction on Monday, June 1, 1996. During this "waiting time," we attended a family wedding at which time I couldn't enjoy myself during this joyous occasion. All I could think about was how my surgery would work out. Being a woman of great faith, I put my faith and trust in God and my doctors who were very conscientious and compassionate.

Due to the stage of my cancer, I didn't require chemotherapy or radiation. I took tamoxifen for five years.

Following my surgery, Carol visited me in the hospital and was very supportive during my recovery. She was in touch with me on a regular basis and invited me to attend a support group with her at her oncologist's office, but I wasn't quite sold on the idea. She persisted and I finally agreed to go. In the end, I was glad that I did. That's where I met an amazing group of women surviving breast cancer and we all had something in common in that we all experienced the same hopes and fears. That's where I became aware of an oncology group for women called Camp Bravehearts. The three co-founders of Camp Bravehearts also attended this support group and were given an opportunity to attend a retreat for women surviving cancer in upstate New York. That spurred their idea of a woman's only oncology retreat that came to fruition in September of 2001, when the first Camp Braveheart retreat was held at Camp Kresge in White Haven, PA. Carol and I went together not knowing what this weekend might bring. And yes, we slept on bunk beds and loved every minute. It brought laughs, tears and an abundance of new friends we could count on through thick and thin. Carol and I attended that first retreat and have been going every year since. Currently Camp Bravehearts offers four retreats a year and is not only for women surviving breast cancer but any cancer, no matter what stage. More information can be found at braveheartscamp.org.

We were eager to meet new friends and share our story in hopes that it could give courage and hope to others on their journey. We also attended Candy's Place, A Cancer Resource Center, which was local to us and was just starting out. We supported Candy's Place and took advantage of the many opportunities that were available to us and we were happy to receive the services offered at no cost to us. And again, a major focus was the opportunity to make new friends along the way.

Prior to the pandemic we were given an opportunity to participate in the YMCA's LiveStrong Program, which is a cancer survivorship program for those who are living with, through, or beyond cancer and is offered at no cost by many YMCA locations. Whoever would have thought that this program would further extend our circle of "cancer friends." Upon completing this program, we were offered the opportunity to attend a Wellness Weekend at of all places, the YMCA's Camp Kresge in White Haven, PA. We went and had the opportunity to meet other survivors who attended previous LiveStrong programs.

We came full circle from 1996 and still counting (28 years for me and 30 years for Carol). Camp Kresge holds a special place in our hearts as well as the hearts of many other cancer survivors and their families.

WHY ME?

BY CAROL MARINO

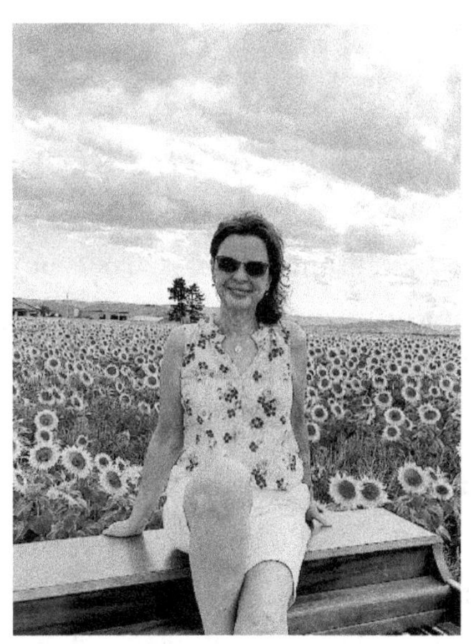

My story began when I married my husband in 1991. As Mona Lisa Vito would say, I was nearing that time of life whereby my (foot-stomping) "biological clock was running out". I did conceive in 1993, however it wasn't in God's plan for us to be parents. So, as a good Catholic girl would do, I prayed for a sign, and I certainly got one. I went for my annual mammogram and got back my "normal' post card in the mail. However, upon a follow-up visit with my gynecologist, a lump was discovered that did not appear on the mammogram. Honestly, I was initially more astonished that it wasn't seen on the mammogram, than the fact I had a lump. A biopsy was needed, and a fine-needle aspiration was done immediately. When that "emergency" was finished, I had my first experience with "waiting." Days passed, while I waited to hear if I would be told those dreaded words or not. When I was called to meet with the doctor, I knew the answer, but I hoped I was wrong. He confirmed the test results and that's when he said those three dreaded words "you have cancer." And there it was, the answer to my questions was that I had breast cancer. I don't know how I got in the car and drove home. I drove to where my husband worked (at a family business) to give him the news. To add more fuel to the fire, my husband had a little red Corvette, and the deal was that when I got pregnant, he'd sell it. He was completing the deal with the buyer when I had to deliver the news. As many other have experienced hearing this news, I put the cart before the horse and had my "end of life" scenario planned out in my head in record time.

The internet then wasn't like it is today and I was afraid to read so I relied on the advice of an aunt who was a well-seasoned, knowledgeable nurse of the day. I didn't know anyone who had been through this; I didn't even know what questions to ask, so I was happy for the advice she gave me. She was spot-on with the referral advice I was given. To this day, I am grateful that the oncologist and surgeon still have me under their watchful eye, most likely because my family has a high rate of cancer. I was very grateful for the plastic surgeon who put me back together again via the Tram-Flap reconstruction, and I was sad to hear of his passing.

News in a small town travels like wild fire, and I got a call from a woman in my hometown who also had been diagnosed with breast cancer and was further along in her treatment process. She was a big help when it came to being prepared for the hair loss I would eventually experience. On the bright side, my wig was always ready to go. I even had more time in the morning before heading off to work, because I didn't need to wash and style. That is, on the days when I felt well enough to work.

My breast cancer was caught early, but it was suggested that due to my young age (42 ½) that I take a round of chemo (4 treatments, 1 month apart). Therefore, in March of 1994 I sat for the first of four treatments. The treatment staff were angels to say the least. With one down and three to go, the next step was "waiting" for my hair to release. But I was prepared. Nausea was a big problem, and the only solace was........wait for it......the biggest, cheesiest, grandest meal that Taco Bell could muster up. I could gag thinking about it today but that's what sustained me. And I made it through.

. . .

My oncologist's office offered a support group for breast cancer survivors, so I hesitantly attended my first meeting in May of 1994. They must have noticed the terrified look on my face because they welcomed me with open arms. As we introduced ourselves, one lady stated she was a seven year survivor. I could only hope and pray that I could someday say the same.

Once I started to rebound after my treatments, I came across a volunteer with the American Cancer Society's Reach to Recovery Program; a program that matches a volunteer with a newly diagnosed breast cancer patient. That's when I realized that no one should have to walk their journey without a support buddy and I knew that my future would involve supporting these women. I was trained by the ACS and began supporting many thankful ladies over many years, and I assisted well over 100 ladies. Many of them are Camp Braveheart sisters and to this day, I am still in touch with the first lady I visited.

I have been blessed throughout my journey with a loving family and supportive friends but never in my wildest dreams did I ever think that having had cancer would bring so many new friends into my life.

The primary reason for this is that Camp Bravehearts brought hundreds of women surviving cancer. More than surviving, they were thriving and living their lives. These ladies supported each other through thick and thin and would be there at the drop of a hat to offer their support. Camp Bravehearts was founded by three young women who were also part of the support group I attended. You can log onto braveheartscamp.org for more information.

In February 2024, it will be thirty years since I heard those three words. There are times that I hesitate to say "30 years" out loud because sometimes "survivor's guilt" comes over me like a wave, but in the end I am truly grateful to be here today to share my story of hope. Having had cancer didn't come wrapped up with a bow but it did come with the blessing of many new, cherished friends, family and a life after having had cancer. Perhaps my survival longevity is the answer to "Why Me" as it allowed me to share my story and my hope with so many others.

DO IT AFRAID!

BY NANCY STEIN

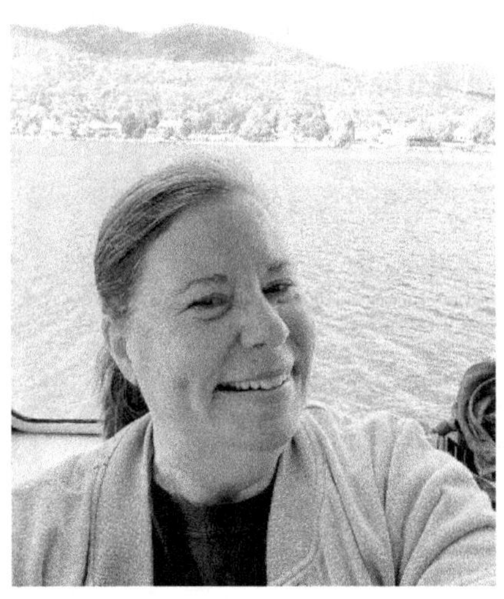

I t was May 20, 2017. My husband was away; a rarity in itself. I watched the Preakness Stakes while enjoying some Italian food and gambling with my cousins via text. After the race, I went to the bathroom and realized that I had just peed blood. A LOT of blood. At the age of 51, I had been in menopause for five months, but just in case it was break-through bleeding, I inserted a tampon, drank a ton of water, waited two hours, then peed again.

Again, a LOT of blood.

I went to the ER. Uncertain of whether or not this consti-tuted an emergency, I asked the triage nurse "I'm peeing blood but there is no pain. Should I be here?" The nurse gulped and said "Oh hell yes. Let me get you right in."

A CT scan was performed, as well as a urinalysis and blood tests. As I waited for the results in the general seating area of our brand-new ER, I looked through the windows and gasped at the incredible sunset that was unfolding in front of me. Due to the light levels, I could also see an excellent reflection of the room I was in, and all that was happening behind me. I casually looked at the reflection of the nurse's station. I saw my nurse, then my doctor. Then I saw more people congregating. Another nurse, another doctor...and was that a social worker? I watched as they began talking intensely. A moment later, they were all looking in my direc-tion. I watched them all approach and decided to make it easier for them.

Before the doctor said a word, I said "Let me do this for you. I don't have a bladder infection."

"No, you do not" replied the doctor.

"I don't have kidney stones."

"No, there are no stones."

I thought for a moment, then said "So you are telling me that I am f^cked."

The doctor barely paused. "You need to see a urologist immediately on Monday morning. Here's a list; get an appointment with the first one who can get you in."

No one said "Cancer." No one had to.

I faced a dilemma; should I tell my husband, who was away on a school music trip? Or should I wait for him to get home late the following night? We had just lost his brother at age 58 to cancer two years previously. His mother had also died at 58 of cancer, when I was pregnant with our first child. I hated to tell him this. However, if I did not tell him, he might be horrified that I had sat with that information alone for 36 hours. I decided to tell him. That was a miserable conversation, but he confirmed what I thought; he was glad I had told him right away, and he did NOT want me struggling alone.

That Monday, we met with a urologist, one of the few kind and gentle ones I have known. He sat and listened as I recounted my ER visit and findings. When I was done, he said "Right. Let's get you scheduled for the correct evaluations." He then rushed from the room, even ordering staff to go to the parking lot to grab the scheduler before she could leave for the day. He raced in and out of offices, getting "first available" on all the testing he wanted. As he paused for a moment in the hall, I said to him, "For the record, I'm very concerned." He looked at me and said "For the record, so am I."

More testing followed, including a cystoscopy two days later. A cystoscopy involves putting a tube roughly the size of a catheter into the urethra, then threading in a camera, to get immediate views of the inner surface of the bladder. The results are projected onto a monitor so the interior of the bladder can be seen by all. As he came into the room to do the test, he said those eight little words everyone hates: "We need to talk about your CAT scan." He had redone the CT with contrast, which the hospital had not used. Without a moment's hesitation, I said, "I have cancer." It was not a question; it was a statement. He replied, "Yes you do. Let me show it to you on the CT and then we will do this test." The CT showed a three-centimeter tumor, which was confirmed by the cystoscopy. How strange it was, to look at the monitor and see this tumor practically waving at me. However, the doctor was quick to reassure me; this was a one-time thing and surgery would be a cure. He was sure it was low grade and would never come back.

The surgeon was called into the room, and he quickly confirmed what we were seeing. He told me that he had a cancellation for the following week; did I want surgery immediately, or did I want to sit and process the information for a while first? I replied, "I would do it today if I could." All presurgical testing was scheduled, and I was able to have my surgery nine days after my first symptom.

This surgery, like every other surgery/checkup/treatment, was done through my urethra. I awoke with a catheter, which was completely unexpected. Unfortunately, I never saw the nice urologist again, as the surgeon had taken over my case. We were sent home with the barest of catheter care instructions for the week, at the end of which the catheter would be removed. I am not squeamish, so I quickly learned how to empty the bag, transition to a night bag, and how to avoid the worst of the intense discomfort. Basically, I had to lay/sit still. Any movement of the catheter would cause severe bladder spasms, which was a new and completely unwelcome sensation. I do wonder how people with no medical background manage their catheter care with no instruction, however.

Back to the "never again, this is a cure!" Nope. I had aggressive bladder cancer that was very likely to return; I was lucky that it was early Stage 1. The pathology was clear; this was not over.

Once I had healed, it was time for treatment. Again, bladder cancer offers a distinct benefit. Because the cancer was on the surface of the inside of my bladder, the treatments were put directly into my bladder via a catheter. On the plus side, the overall effects from the treatments were muted. I didn't get badly sick or lose my hair. The downside was that I had to be catheterized constantly, which is not something the urethra is comfortable with. For my first treatment, I was taken into a large space in which there were six beds, surrounded by flimsy curtains. As I was being escorted to my "room," I noticed that of course the curtains were not fully closed, and I had the unwelcome ability to see a lot of men naked from the waist down. I froze and requested a private room. When I was asked why, I replied "I do not wish to see naked men, and the fact that I can see them means that they can see me, and I do not consent to that!" I was "reassured" that only the medical people would be able to see me (present penises excepted), and they were "comfortable seeing naked people." I replied "I don't care what they are comfortable seeing! I care what I'm comfortable showing, and I'm not comfortable exposing myself."

Not surprisingly, a side room was found. It's amazing to me that I had to ask more than once.

I was scheduled to have six initial treatments, once a week for six weeks. When I came for the second treatment, the doctor was unavailable so the nurse did it. Imagine my surprise when she used numbing gel in my urethra before using the catheter! It made such a difference with regard to my comfort. The following week, the doctor was back. I asked him why he didn't use numbing gel. His answer: "You are a woman, so your urethra is shorter than a man's, so it doesn't hurt you AS MUCH" (my emphasis added). I stared at him until he gulped, then I slowly said "Let me make sure I have this clear. You had the means to lessen my pain, but you made a unilateral decision NOT to do that, without offering it to me, even though it would be at no cost or extra effort for you???" He stared at the floor and mumbled "Yes Ma'am." I waited a few more moments, then said "Do you know that thing that you've been doing to your female patients without discussing with them? DO NOT DO THAT TO ANYONE EVER AGAIN."

This practice made me nervous because they did not think I needed maintenance treatments. By then, I had done a tremendous amount of reading of research articles, and they were all clear; high grade disease is high risk. I transferred to a larger medical center, which had a doctor who specialized in bladder cancer. Unfortunately, he was a grumpy old man, prone to grumbling and with no social skills whatsoever. At the time, I was also wrestling with Medical PTSD, which is no joke. I have a history of being assaulted when I was giving birth to my first child (VERY long story short; the OB and the midwife were in the middle of a nasty argument when I started pushing, and the OB decided to take her aggression and frustration out on my body, which led to a hip-to-hip crash C-section when the baby's heart stopped), so having to have so much traffic in my privates was incredibly alarming to me. And just as predicted by everyone but my first team, my cancer came right back three months after my initial cancer. Back to surgery, back to catheters, back to treatment.

Realizing that this cancer would be a part of my life for a long time, if not forever, pushed me into therapy to try to cope. At the time, all I was feeling was anger, and I was stuck there. With the help of an excellent therapist who specialized in Women's Trauma, I was able to move on, even as the cancer came back two additional times after the first recurrence. I'm now with Memorial Sloan Kettering, and I'm finally comfortable with a team. The doctor is great, and so are the nurses.

As I began my research for retreats for women with cancer, I was disappointed to find that most opportunities are for women who have breast cancer. Breast cancer is seen in roughly a third of all new female cancers in a given year, and receives approximately 12% of all cancer funding. Breast cancer receives ten times more funding than the 12 next most common cancers combined. Bladder cancer is typically seen in old men who smoke and drink, none of which describes me. This discrepancy helped me to see a need and become the administrator for a Facebook page for women with bladder cancer. We are an international group and I have moderators in each time zone. At present, we have over 2600 members.

The most upsetting part of this cancer is the knowledge that bladder cancer is underreported in women. In my Facebook group, if a woman presents with Stage 3-4 right from the beginning, I can be pretty certain that the delay in diagnosis (leading to a miserable outcome at this level) was due to being ignored or condescended to by doctors. I am on a crusade to tell women (and remind doctors!) that if a woman pees blood, CHECK FOR BLADDER CANCER.

At my second recurrence, I found myself needing a break. I was just so depleted. My husband and two adult children were great about everything, but my mom seemed angry and dismissive. My dad was unwell. There was a great deal of pressure on me. I decided to try to find a retreat for women who had cancer. I located a retreat weekend being hosted by Camp Good Days and Special Times, on Keuka Lake NY. And then, I froze. How could I go alone to a group of about 60 women? How could I sleep in a cabin with strangers? Then I reminded myself; Do It Afraid. To me, this means to do things that are scary, because I probably don't have a very long life span in front of me. I need to assume things will work out. I ask myself, what is the worst thing that could happen, and how will I handle it? I gave myself permission to stay in a motel or Airbnb if I felt uncomfortable. Then, I WENT. And I was so glad I did!

I made such wonderful friends who laughed with me, goofed off with me, and cried with me. Everyone was wonderful, including the staff. I was able to go back two times before Covid had us all tucked up in our homes.

A friend from Camp Good Days told me about another camp, Camp Bravehearts. Again I applied, and again my brain began catastrophizing. So again, I did it anyway. I did it afraid.

Once again, I met the most amazing women. I made friends quickly and came to love this group, especially the founders, who had been "in the trenches" in their own lives. I have gone to Bravehearts three times, and each one has been amazing, with different activities, as well as different moments of clarity, pain, and love.

As of this writing, I have had high grade/aggressive bladder cancer four times in just under seven years. We have beat it back each time, but so far I've had to endure four surgeries, approximately 20 cystoscopies, and 57 treatments. All this, while working part to full time as a Speech Language Pathologist in private practice. I've just finished another round of treatment, and if there is no sign of cancer during my next check in two months, I will re-enter a three-year sequence of three treatments every three months, cystoscopies once every three months, for three years. I've accepted that as the best-case scenario, and I no longer live in anger. Having other women who understand the cancer merry-go-round, even if our disease is in different parts of our bodies, has helped tremendously. I don't want people to think that we just sit around and cry. Much more typical is the sound of our laughter. I'm so fortunate to be with others who are "doing it afraid" and living their best lives. I strongly recommend that everyone "do it afraid." Life is limited, so don't have regrets.

FEAR TO GROWTH

BY KAREN CATALANO

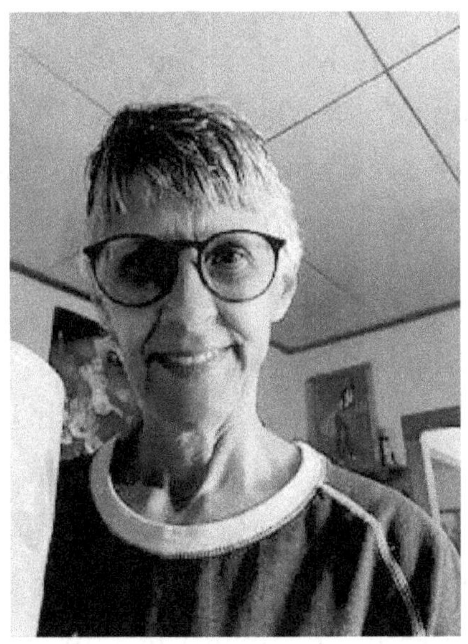

When others were thinking about the Christmas season and all its light, I felt distraught because I was being tested for an abnormality in my right breast. I could not concentrate well to pull off the season that I am usually so excited for. This was distressing me as I received bad vibes from my personal physician.

I had undergone getting my gall bladder out in October. It went well, and I saw the surgeon who had performed the operation prior to my own discovery of an unusual lump as I checked out my laparoscopic scars from the gallbladder surgery. I had been instructed as par for the course to see my general physician as a continued follow-up regarding the gallbladder. Things looked good to him, which I was pleased. When I got up from the examining table, I asked my doctor if he wouldn't mind checking out the lump I discovered. He immediately said, "Oh Karen, I don't like this. I am sending you to the hospital for further checking." He got right on the phone and called for who he wanted me to see to set up an appointment.

At that point right there, I felt I was doomed. My doctor had such an expression on his face and tone to his voice that I knew he had previous experience with this. I first had an appointment for an ultrasound, and the doctor who would be dealing with me was called in during the ultrasound. He looked and said. "This will need to be biopsied." Oh geez, now I had two doctors who confirmed my fear. Within a few days, I had the biopsy done on that particular lump and an additional mass on the other side the doctor discovered.

When he took out the piece he was after, he took on a tone of great sensitivity with me, as he could tell it was malignant right then and there. This was happening just a couple days before Christmas. He said it would take a few days for the results and with it being a holiday weekend, he warned we that might not know the results until after Christmas which was Monday. He told me that results should be back on the 26th. Then he quietly added, "Now Mrs. Catalano, I would like you to come back to me for the surgery to take care of this." He placed his hand on my shoulder which was confirming in my mind that he knew it was malignant.

Those few days were so long and draining for me. I had to act like I was so happy that it was Christmas and a season of blessings. I prayed and prayed. My daughter was home from college, and my husband worked his normal schedule, having off Christmas Eve and Christmas Day. I just acted like life was going on as planned, but my heart was broken and a thousand thoughts rushed in my head - I have a daughter, and a husband, and other family members I cared deeply for. I worked a full-time job and worked those last days before that holiday weekend. All along from what was Thanksgiving to Christmas was hell knowing that I may have cancer and the future had many uncertainties. My head spun. I thought this cannot be, this cannot be happening, maybe the doctors will be wrong, maybe I'm okay and all this fussing will be for nothing. Something else bothered me though - why is there seemingly so much time between tests.

Time was ticking and I'm waiting to find out my fate. I really wasn't a "why me" person, yet I knew I always was doing the healthy things for myself. I exercised daily. I didn't drink. I didn't smoke. I ate healthy. There were others who went on to say to me, "Karen, why you? You do everything right. You are too young for this." I guess I had to ask myself how this happened to me. But, as much as those things were true, my fear was about to turn into reality. This is where a person starts seriously thinking that life is unfair.

On December 26th, I called my general doctor for the results, but I was met with "we've not received anything yet Karen. Can you call later this afternoon?" Well, later that afternoon, my daughter came with me to the office as I wanted to check in with them in person. The nurse said, "Oh hold on, we have something sitting in the fax machine." She walked back out with that fax while I was standing out in the hall. She continued, "Karen, your results are here, I'm sorry, but the finding is indicating malignancy. Let me get the doctor for you." We were all on friendly terms as I knew these folks, so the nurse was free to tell me what she read. And my doctor was at the end of his day with patients, and came out to the hall. He began with "Hello Megan (my daughter), you're as beautiful as ever, how is college going?" He then turned to me and said "Karen, your lump was as suspected, what do you want to do from here? You can go back to the doctor who did the biopsy as he would like to do your surgery. Or there is the cancer center in Dubois." I knew there was the cancer center and thought that would be my best choice. I said I want to go there, what do I need to do? He said "We will get this info over there for you and they will call you with your next step."

Being that my 19 year old daughter was with me, I knew immediately that I was taking the bravest front I ever had to do. I knew I wanted to be there for her, and my husband and family. This diagnosis was not going to get me down. I had done all my worrying with my worst fears in November through December of 2006. December 26 was my day to turn this into an experience of positivity. My fear had come true, so now I knew I must get beyond that and move forward. Now my thoughts were on getting through the next steps, while keeping my chin up.

The next day I received a call from Hahne Cancer Center in Dubois about seeing me as soon as possible, and I was set up with a wonderful surgeon, Dr. P, the day after New Years. She made me feel like this would all be fine. That day was all about doing her own tests and having me talk to people in social work who let me know what would be available to me should I or any family members need it. I came home with pamphlets covering everything from what is cancer, what to expect in treatments depending on final diagnosis, to how to pick out a wig, and if needed, how to choose a prosthetic. It was overwhelming, intimidating and yet comforting. They made this all so less scary. Having direction sure helped me. These people had my best interests at heart. My family, of which I will include my work family, also had my best interest at heart. A strong support system helps us survive. I was so lucky to have that. That time frame went so fast compared to what I had experienced with the initial tests in November and December. I didn't have time to feel sorry for myself, nor did I want to. I had even told Dr. P I want both breasts removed, then I would not have to worry about having that happen again (although I certainly knew about a recurrences or metastasis). She would not do that though, as she thought this would be devastating enough. I still wish she had though at that time, because I wound up having to have the second breast removed a few years later.

Doctor P did a right mastectomy and removed 3-4 lymph nodes. Then I was set up for a full treatment regimen. This was confusing to me because I had older neighbors and a close older friend who had breast cancer at the same time as me didn't have all that. They each had only removal of the indicated lump, and one had chemotherapy and the others had only radiation. I had the full scale of treatment - mastectomy, chemo, and radiation, and had my ovaries removed after treatment as I had an estrogen positive cancer. They said it was standard protocol to treat mine fully as I was considered young and they wanted to see me live a fuller life. Now these women lived full lives, in fact two are still alive and in their 90's. I pray to be as lucky as those gals.

I did experience a couple of setbacks early in my treatment. After the surgery to remove my breast, I recovered well, three weeks later had my port put in, and then had my first chemo cocktail in mid February. It was certainly a humbling experience but had been a much better experience than what I expected. Yes, I was queasy, but given great anti nausea meds, and tired, but given time to rest, and a Neulasta shot to counteract the damage of the chemo, as we know chemo kills good cells with bad cells. But then wham...I was so sick and could not even get up from the bathroom floor. I was scared out of my mind, and my husband more than I.

We were to call Hahne with anything that I needed to report or question. My husband made that call, and there I was thinking the chemo was doing just what I had truly feared - the constant nausea we saw in old movies that people suffered. I was devastated in my mind, thinking "I can't do this. I'm going to die trying to stay alive. Oh my God help me." There is one thing I cannot stand and that is being nauseated. Never could, and never will. Hahne went through the timeline of my chemo day, my nausea meds for 3 days to follow, the Neulasta shot, and stated it's not the chemo making you that sick. What?? They wanted to see me, so the only way to go was by ambulance to the ER in Dubois. My mind raced thinking how did this go so bad so quick. I was trying so hard to be positive and come out of this just fine.

The ER staff was very attentive to my needs. They took vitals, labs, the usual. Oh my, the panic buttons went off for them in short order with the labs. I don't remember just how many nurses ran into that ER room, but I couldn't see any one of the four walls. They said "Your counts are off the chart, you have something awful going on, perhaps a secondary cancer." Oh dear God. As soon as they said it was my blood counts that were sky high, I said "I had the Neulasta shot yesterday." That was omitted in stating the timeline of the treatment I had in previous days to them (I assumed they knew that as my oncology team called them to say I was coming). Wow, they breathed a sigh of relief that was actually heard by everyone in the room - an actual "WHEW". The doctor said "oh thank God for that, as now we know why your counts are high. But, we don't know what is happening to you." So I was admitted for further evaluation, in isolation for them to figure out what was making me so incredibly sick. It took one special ER doctor who did some "petri dish" studies to figure out 3 days later what was making me so ill. He came in my room in an isolation suit and mask, as all the nurses and doctors did and he said "We know what is making you so ill; it's C diff." It was my 50th birthday. Here I was stuck in a room by myself with no visitors allowed no birthday cake, feeling like a leper. I was bummed to say the least, and I didn't feel good either. My hero doctor explained to me what C diff was, because I didn't know. Then he asked "Do you want the good news or the bad news?" "The good news please" I replied. He said "The good news is it is treatable and there are two meds we could use." I said "Great!" He said, "Well now for the bad news, one is Flagyl and the other is Vancomycin." I was allergic to Flagyl which was the bad news. "So," he continued, "we must hope the vancomycin will be good for you. If it doesn't work, we will have to send you somewhere else." So, we went with the vancomycin and I was kept another day and God blessed me and it worked. Eighteen days of pills that totally did the trick to rid of the C diff and I felt so much better almost immediately.

When I went for a check up with my oncologist after my hospital visit and prior to my second chemo visit, my oncologist said it was up to me, but due the circumstances of how sick I got, that it might not be in my best interest to continue with chemo. I said …no, no. I am to get four rounds of chemo, I want to beat this! Dr. M was well known for using his many sources of other physicians. He said, "Let me make a phone call." I was getting adriamycin as part of my "cocktail" as they called it and that was likely to have been the drug that caused me to get the C diff. It is potent stuff. He stepped out of the office and came back while I talked to my husband and a couple of family members who were in attendance with me. We all were shocked that I was advised not to get further chemo. I said I'm not happy to have to stop the chemo, and no, I don't want C diff again, but geez. I think I did have tears in my eyes then as I was thinking in the back of my mind, "How can I win this battle now, how can I be around to be here for my daughter, my husband Jim, my family." When Dr. M came back in the room he said, "I have a plan for you Karen, we will change up your meds in the chemo, remove the adriamycin replacing it with taxotere." He told me the possible effects of taking taxotere, and if I got that ill again, then we would have to stop. I said, "I am in!! I want 4 of those if they work out." He said, "You only need 3, as we see now, that first one did what it was supposed to do. It killed the good cells with the bad cells, and that is the primary reason we use chemotherapy drugs for cancer. To get to all the bad cells, and in the process it of course kills good cells. for you Karen…it worked." I said "I still want 4 of the same." He finally agreed, and I had 4 treatments of the new cocktail without incident. Thank God. I went back to chemo a couple of weeks later while he said I would recuperate better from having the C diff.

I had lost my hair before I got to the second treatment. I expected that. As it started to fall out in clumps, I was back working and my fellow workers were very saddened as to what they saw, one of my friends there cried and cried. I went to my hairdresser very soon after that and had her shave my head, and my husband shaved his too. My next stop was to get a wig and a few doo rags. Doo rags were fun! All kinds of fun designs. The wig was hard to choose as I didn't find any that were like my hair style which really was a simple shoulder length bob and jet black in color. I choose a style that was a deep dark brown and had not quite the same length and a bit of bangs. Of course, what happened was a bit hurtful to my spirit. I went to work, and my coworkers were absolutely great in helping me, I only had to sit at my desk and do my paperwork and they took care of the customers. That first morning was a busy one with a full lobby of folks (I worked in a bank) and one guy hollered from the end station "Hey, hey, what did you do to your hair?" Oh, I didn't even want to look up when I heard him. Every customer in the lobby was staring at me. The girls around me came to my rescue and had my boss call me to the back room so I could escape that situation. One of them went and talked to the customer who really was a nice man, but he caused such a scene. A couple of women I worked with were so upset and crying; I didn't cry, but it sure made me self-conscious about that damn wig, but I wasn't going to work in a doo rag or a bald head. I just quietly let people know I was in treatment, and the word spread. As I said, I live in a small town. What are you going to do?

I must tell a story here about how I eased my concerns about my hairless head. Hopefully it helps anyone out there who felt like I did about losing my hair. It truly bothered me more than losing my breast. No one was going to know about that, but I couldn't hide that something affected my hair suddenly.

It was getting to be spring at this point of the events - March into April, and the weather was getting very nice. I had always been a walker, and I sure had an itch to go walking at the track at the high school which is my favorite place to walk. My husband joined me as he wasn't going to let me go by myself the first time in case I didn't feel well. We were walking, and it was just lovely outside, but I was getting warm, and I felt the head- covering doo rag was too warm to be wearing but didn't want to remove it. I was kind of struggling with that. As we were walking, a woman came up from behind us. She was in a two-piece jogging suit, it was a pale gray and had a pink stripe running down each leg, and a pink stripe on each arm length. Her hair was brown and styled very nice, wavy, going just past her shoulders. I could not see her face as she jogged by us. She said, "Oh honey, just take that off your head, I've been there. Let it go." I was trying to figure out who this lady was, but I took off that rag immediately as it was a true relief to do so. I knew everyone who seemed to use the track but I had never seen this woman. My husband asked, "who was that?" I said "I don't know, I never saw her before." We looked out ahead of us and she was not in front of us, and we looked behind us, and to the other side of the track. That woman vanished as quickly as it seemed she came from nowhere to be on the track. There were only two ways open to the track at the time. How she came on and how she left that track so quickly was a puzzle to us both. I, as well as my husband, to this day think she was an angel to comfort me in the particular struggle I was feeling with the hair loss. After that day, I was never concerned with my hair or lack of it. I did wear the wig when working at the bank, but other times I went to town or appointments with a doo rag or just a ball hat. An angel for me, wow. How could I think otherwise?

I have another story to share about my journey, as the C diff issue was troubling to myself and family, and the chemo causes some lousy days the first week of every chemo treatment. My dear mother-in-law was so upset that I would be ill or in pain and she came up to see me one day. In my house the great conversation place is my kitchen table. We sat down there as she wanted to tell me how awful she felt that I was suffering. I assured her that what I was feeling was to be expected, that the second week after chemo was a recovery week and the third week before my next treatment I would feel pretty well. Here I must tell you that my mother-in-law is a very straight laced "politically correct" woman, but with huge compassion, and great kindness and always helpful. She started to tear up and gently crying and saying to me, "Karen, let us take you to Canada and get you some of that marijuana to help you endure this phase of the journey." Oh …all to my surprise, I would never think of this coming out of her. Totally unexpected to think that she would even think this way. I am also very straight laced, and I would not even think to try that. I said that I didn't want to try that, and thanks, but we are not doing anything of the sort. I reassured her I would be okay, and so far so good. It was 2007 when I had a year of surgeries, chemo and radiation. I did okay without marijuana. The doctors and nurses had my back.

Another hilarious story to share, as I laughed the moment it happened. I loved being outdoors working in the yard. One day after work, I felt like weeding and picking up sticks, edging the yard, so I put on my shorts and t shirt and proceeded outside. Now I must tell you I had a prosthetic that was to be able to adhere to my chest if I chose not to wear it in the mastectomy bra. I wanted to try that as it was a warm day. Out the door I went with my newfound freedom of not wearing a bra. Being outside in the warm air was terrific, and I was enjoying my yard work, until I bent over and the prosthetic fell out of the top of my shirt onto the ground. My thoughts were immediately "Who saw that happen!" as I was laughing and picking it up off the ground, and off to the house I went to get a bra on. That was the only day I tried that. God forbid it happened at work or anywhere else. So much for that! I have since had my left breast removed in 2016 just because I was tired of constant biopsies. They took a lot of my fear away that I had from the start as I had wanted my surgeon to remove that breast with the one that was diseased. Now I have two prosthetic breasts. I feel I cannot go without wearing something as I'm not comfortable being totally flat, even though I was never well endowed. I have some pride, and I never want someone to be shocked looking at me. I never considered getting implants, as that sounded painful, and more scars on my body. Nope. Two mastectomies were enough scars.

I guess looking back at this history of my treatment, I had more fear than I realized. I took a lot in stride as you have little time to think and rehashing it has brought back some ugly moments of the whole thing and some good ones also. I can think of the friends I have made through the years that got cancer and how we can talk about it and be okay. Being in the company of others who have experienced the same fears, illness, effects from it (and there are effects of treatment) have all impacted me and in good ways. There was one older man I enjoyed talking to at pretty much every radiation appointment that I had, as we were on much the same schedule. He was a trucker, gruff looking, but so humbled by his experience with throat cancer. He wanted to tell everyone he met that they should never smoke or chew tobacco as he had for many years. He wanted people to learn from his experience. He had terrible burns on his neck from the radiation and lost a small part of his jaw to remove the cancerous part. I felt sorry for him that everyone could see his open wounds, as you could not see what I had done because I could wear clothing to cover it. He was a gentle soul despite his gruff appearance. So easy to talk to, so open with what happened to him. I had my husband come with me one day to meet him as this fellow was a gem to talk to. These are the kind of people I have met on my journey. It has been a raw journey, humbling, depressing, uplifting, a learning experience with my fellow humans. I would not trade any of it that has happened. But I know I have made it so far, and I know many don't do as well as I have. That's the sad part of cancer or any illness that can suck the life out of you - literally.

Having cancer made me stronger, I know that, I feel that. There are days though that it's okay to say I'm tired and I don't want to go through "what doesn't kill you makes you stronger." It's okay to feel vulnerable, to reach out for help, to pray for wellness.

Having cancer taught me to accept that there is really only so much time and that it can be taken for granted. One day at a time is so true as a survivor. No one is promised tomorrow will come. I always have had a bucket list, a grocery list, a list of projects for the house, the car, a list of crafts I wish to complete, something always in my Amazon shopping cart. That hasn't changed for me, but I know that one day I may be ill again with something and none of those lists will matter. I have learned for myself and seeing it with loved ones and friends that you have nothing if you don't have your health. Please live each day as it could be your last. Be kind, be caring, and understanding to others who struggle and comfort them as best you can no matter what kind of illness or issue they have. Be there for them.

I wrote a book recently just because I have wanted to do that for about 20 years. It is a book of family recipes I penned to share with others. I feel that was my biggest bucket list thing and after settling in a few months after retirement to get cracking on it. I had handwritten one for my daughter when she was getting ready to finish up college and get married. I used that book as the basis for mine that I recently compiled. It is a treasure of family recipes to honor my Mom and Grandmother mostly as they were so influential to me in my love of the kitchen and I wanted for others to know they were fabulous strong women. What was neat about this book was I added photos of my second love of artistic expression that I had started a dozen years ago. Crafts, mostly painting I did on pallets, furniture of sorts, bricks, and also a dabbling of some other things. This spin was exposing myself even more than what happened when I had cancer. I will tell you it was something that I was so pleased to share with others. It will hopefully be a bit of myself left behind as I hoped I made a difference in the world I live in.

Anyone who has ever wanted to talk to me about my experience with cancer - I am all in and an open book. I want people to learn from me, to help make a difference, if it helps them to know that they are never alone in that battle, (as you could feel alone). Please know that you all have someone in your corner, watching your back, to be with you, or to pray with you. The power of prayer was a huge asset in my favor and I will never forget those who prayed for me, or prayed for my family not to suffer while I was. The people I met in my journey will never be forgotten by me. They all offered words of wisdom or kind words, caring words, or a caring look in their eyes. Please know as you are reading this, if you want to talk about your innermost fears…I am here for you. You can reach out to almost any survivor. We will listen, we will cry with you, we will laugh with you, we can empathize with you. Been there done that. We each have varied experiences, but if one person learns something from any one of us, we leave a positive mark on this earth. That's what I want to do in so many ways. God put me here, and I'm using that to better myself, and that has become a means to help any other person out there who needs a listening ear, a hug, or a prayer.

I have been blessed in many ways. There has been great love in my life from family and friends. I have had great glory of my own at times that put me on top of the world, and glory from family members who I treasure. That have brought me much joy and pride. I value my family that I love dearly. I am here to know it every day! My bottom-line words are to share, help, love and be kind. Be positive. ;) Grow through your experience. I did.

Love ya, Karen

CDH – WON

BY KALI HERZOG

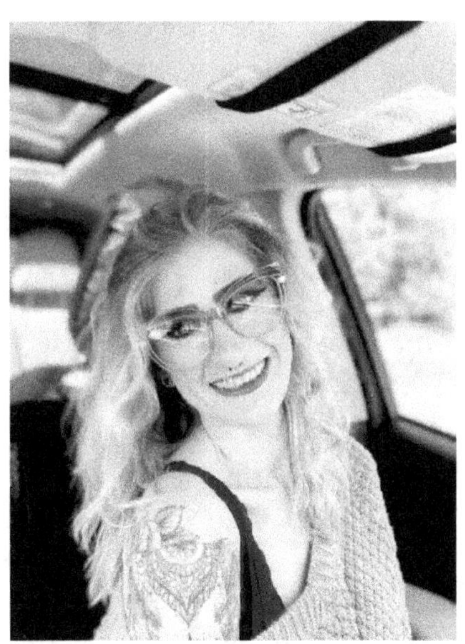

Reflecting on the year 2020, it commenced as a pinnacle in my life but concluded as a formidable challenge. At the age of 23, I found myself assuming new roles as a mother, a successful nurse, a partner, and an independent individual. The initial months were marked by a sense of liberation and self-sufficiency that comes with living independently.

During my pursuit of a nursing education, I qualified for advanced placement, allowing me to commence my studies in December instead of the typical August start. On my inaugural day of nursing school, December 3rd, a significant event unfolded – my mother underwent a stomach removal procedure due to an uncommon CDH1 gene mutation. This mutation, following an autosomal dominant inheritance pattern, involves a germline mutation, meaning a parent with the gene mutation has a 50% chance of passing it on to their child. The CDH1 gene mutation elevates the risk of hereditary diffuse stomach cancer and lobular breast cancer substantially. The prevalence of these cancers is relatively low, with an estimated 1% of the U.S. population developing any type of stomach cancer, and only a fraction of that percentage constituting hereditary diffuse gastric cancer.

Remarkably, the identification of the CDH1 gene mutation occurred in 1998, shedding light on its lethal nature and the associated poor prognosis once diagnosed. My mother, unfortunately, faced the challenge of battling both stomach and breast cancers. Despite the grim statistics, she triumphed over these adversities, emerging as a survivor and my cherished confidante.

I used to joke, "I'm not getting my death sentence in my 20s!" because my mom was adamant I get tested and I didn't want to. It was funny... Until it wasn't....

Upon discovering my pregnancy and contemplating the responsibilities that motherhood would entail, I recognized the importance of taking the necessary steps. The genetic testing occurred when my son reached 11 months, when I was 23, with my 24th birthday approaching in a month. The process involved providing a saliva sample in a small container, a seemingly prolonged endeavor. Anticipating the results within two weeks, I approached the appointment optimistically, free from significant worry.

During the subsequent appointment, the unexpected news echoed – I tested positive for the gene mutation. The shock was palpable, and the details shared by the doctor became a blur in my overwhelmed state. Alone in a small white room, tears flowed as I grappled with the reality unfolding before me.

Swiftly, I was scheduled with a GI Doctor at UPMC Shadyside, embarking on an endoscopy (EGD). The doctor, who coincidentally had treated my mother, brought a comforting familiarity to the situation. Despite his shorter stature, his kindness, sweetness, and gentle demeanor played a crucial role. The procedure involved the extraction of 60 biopsies, with the promise of results in a week.

Two days later, January 8th, at 6:30 pm, no one else was home, and I got a call from a Pittsburgh number. I didn't think anything of it because it was evening time and it had only been two days since my EGD, and results were not due for a week.

It was my doctor… "Kali, I'm sorry to tell you this but you have cancer. 26/60 of the biopsies tested positive for cancer." I was shattered, scared, heartbroken, in denial; a ton of emotions. All I remember saying to him was "Can you call my dad?" I was a sobbing mess and scared to death. Plus I had just turned 24 years old. WTF. Who gets cancer that young? I tried to gather myself enough to call my dad, the conversation was short. We were both so shocked neither one of us knew what to say. I honestly don't even remember how I told my mom or sisters. I was so sick over telling my mom because I didn't want her to feel any guilt.

I was referred to an oncologist at UPMC Presby. My dad and I went to my appointment together. It was an easy decision to tell the doctor I wanted my stomach removed and I asked him to schedule me ASAP. I knew that I was going to have a tough road ahead of me, but I had no clue of the severity it was going to be. This was also during the pandemic, so you could only have one support person with you at your appointments. It wasn't an easy decision to pick my support person, but after a lot of time and consideration, my dad ended up being my support person. We decided that we were going to keep me having cancer as a secret because Elk

County, where I was living, is a small community and we didn't want people to know our business. Plus, this was devastating news, and I didn't want my "friends" or people who were nosey to reach out to me about it. I wasn't prepared to hear "I'm sorry" or "if you need anything…" just to be let down because no one would follow through.

On January 26, my baby had just turned one four days earlier and I was about to have a major surgery. I made a video of myself the day before my surgery, the day of, and a couple times afterwards. Now it's 2024 and I haven't watched all of them yet because I'm just not ready. The nurses and doctor told my dad it would be about 3 and a half hours for my procedure. That wasn't bad timing since I was getting my entire stomach removed. 8 HOURS LATER, I was finally out of surgery. There were complications such as finding out that the cancer had spread to my intestines and my esophagus. They had to remove a section of my intestines and a section of my esophagus. They did this because they wanted to verify that they successfully eliminated the cancer cells to deter further cancer growth. I had drains, I had cuts, I had pain, and I had no idea what I was about to endure as my new life was beginning.

When I was in the hospital, they tried a feeding tube. My body wouldn't take it. I would immediately throw up or get diarrhea. We tried the feeding tube too many times to count. They ultimately ended up putting me on TPN (Total parenteral nutrition) for twelve hours a day which consisted of being hooked up to an IV that contained the nutrients I needed because I was unable to eat. I had to relearn how to eat food entirely, and to this day I am still trying to figure out what my body can and cannot tolerate. I would joke around and say that my son and I were eating purees at the same time. The first day I came home from the hospital, I tried to eat a pizza lunchable because I was convinced I could eat regular food and the doctor was just being cautious. WRONG. It was a nightmare, and I was so sad I couldn't eat something so small. I remember I would put food in my mouth and chew it just to get the taste, and then having to spit it out so I wouldn't choke or vomit.

I spent the next six months on complete bed rest. I was hooked up to TPN every single night for twelve hours. If I had to pee, I had to pause it or if I wanted to move, I had to pause it, and that just prolonged the process so I always tried to not move because I wanted it to just be over. I would have to lay flat on my back, with my arm extended because my port was on my upper right arm. I didn't get to hold my son for an entire year, that was probably the hardest thing. I tried to work when I could, but because of my health I am still unemployed. I would spend most of my days binge watching Law and Order: SVU, crying, having accidents, or being fed by "Big Bertha," which is what we named the TPN bags to lighten the situation. Plus, it looked like a big bag of white milk and the name just fit. Before surgery I was 138 pounds. I instantly started dropping weight. My lowest was 98 pounds. Right now, I hover between 110-115. Community nurses would come in two or three times a week. I always hated having a younger nurse because I was so young, and I almost felt embarrassed. I finally got a nurse that I had known for many years, and she took care of me so well. She lectured when she had to and laughed with me while I would sit with tears in my eyes as she was changing my port.

Despite this horrific "recovery," I was determined more than ever to get better.

Because of having gastric cancer, it was inevitable that at some point in my life I was going to get breast cancer. I opted to get a prophylactic bilateral mastectomy with reconstruction at the beginning of 2022. This surgery was more devastating than the cancer because I literally felt like I was losing a part of what made me a woman. I still feel that way today. I had drains on both of my sides that would drain fluid from my incision site. I'd have to track how much fluid was in my drain and record it every time I emptied them. I felt so disgusted with my body and betrayed. How could this possibly have happened? What did I do so wrong? This is a question I face every single day. I am still struggling but pushing through. Leaning on our community has now become my life, and it stinks having to ask for help that because of my cancer I am now so strapped with doctors almost every day, infusions three times a week over an hour away from my hometown, B12 injections weekly, still vomiting and having accidents. Fighting every day to get out of bed, praying I will not be sick. I'm so tired of being sick. My poor son has been such a trooper, he is one special kid.

Since being diagnosed with cancer up until now, I have been hospitalized over 20 times due to this disease.

While having cancer really sucked and some days I wanted to really give up, it has taught me three valuable life lessons: Hope, Resilience, and Acceptance.

Hope:

Having cancer is a life-altering experience that transformed the very core of my existence. The initial shock and fear gave way to a profound sense of vulnerability, forcing me to confront the fragility of life. In the midst of physical and emotional turmoil, unexpected sources of hope emerged. The journey through cancer taught me resilience, fostering a newfound appreciation for the precious moments and relationships that often go unnoticed in the hustle of everyday life. Each day became a triumph, a testament to the strength within. The support of loved ones, the resilience of the human spirit, and advancements in medical science fueled my hope. Despite the challenges, I found a renewed purpose and a deeper connection to the resilience that exists within us all. Cancer, in its darkest moments, became a catalyst for transformation, ultimately illuminating the power of hope to guide me and my family through the most challenging chapters of our lives. But, with time, I slowly gained hope for healing, and I have held on to this since day one.

Resilience:

Facing cancer was a radical change in my life, a journey marked by both physical and emotional distress. The diagnosis plunged me into an unfamiliar realm of uncertainty and vulnerability. Yet, within the crucible of adversity, I discovered an unexpected reservoir of resilience. The challenges, treatments, and uncertainties served as crucibles that tested the nerve of my spirit. Each setback became an opportunity to cultivate strength, perseverance, and an unyielding determination to confront the formidable foe that is cancer. I worked hard every single day. Trying new foods, keeping my weight up, going to Pittsburgh every week for months. The experience taught me that resilience is not the absence of adversity, but rather the ability to adapt and thrive in its presence. As I navigated the arduous path of fighting this battle, I found solace in the unwavering support of loved ones and the courage within myself. Cancer became a teacher, imparting lessons of tenacity, gratitude for each day, and an enduring belief in the resilience that resides within the human spirit.

Acceptance:

The journey through cancer was a profound transformation that reshaped my perspective on life, instilling in me the virtue of acceptance. Initially met with disbelief and resistance, I gradually learned to embrace the reality of my diagnosis and the uncertainties that lay ahead. I knew if I had a negative mindset, I'd never get better. It wasn't and still isn't easy to give up the stability I had. I live in a world now of constant chaos, time never slowing down. Doctors' appointments almost every day. I have come to accept this is my new life and just because I did what I had to do, doesn't necessarily mean I am comfortable in my emotions but at the end of the day, I have accepted what has and is to come. Cancer forced me into a space of where I had to surrender, where I had to accept the ups and downs of the journey, the unpredictability of treatment outcomes, and the impermanence of life itself. This acceptance was not a resignation to fate, but a conscious choice to find peace amongst the chaos. It involved acknowledging the vulnerability of my own body and understanding that healing was not only physical but also a mental and emotional process. Hell, I'm still healing. Through the highs and lows, acceptance became a powerful ally, allowing me to navigate the challenges with a sense of grace and serenity. In the face of misfortune, I discovered that true strength lies not just in resistance but in the ability to accept, adapt, and find meaning in the midst of life's most profound challenges.

At the end of the day, no matter how hard it is, I thank God for keeping me alive. Having a 15% chance of survival is a scary thing to go through, and it's even more scary when you have a precious, innocent child who must endure all your struggles with you. He handles it well, and even if he doesn't fully understand he accepts what is and I am proud that he is still able to learn and read and laugh and enjoy life despite mommy always being sick.

My advice to someone with cancer? Sounds cliche, but don't give up. Stay positive. Do you have kids? Keep them at the forefront. Days are going to really suck, and that's okay. No one expects you to have a good day every day. Take time for yourself. This is something I still struggle with, but I am working on it. It has taken me years to accept my prognosis, but I am learning to accept it. Someday you will too. Remember, cancer doesn't define you. It teaches you valuable life lessons that you didn't even realize you needed or lacked. Always lean on God. My cancer journey brought me closer to him. I talk to him daily now and he knows all my emotions. He knows when I'm happy, sad, mad, pissed, glad, thankful. He knows before I even do. And my last piece of advice, keep your family close. Lean on them, especially in your darkest times. They will guide you through, and help you get through your journey. I won't lie, it's a horrible path, but it's also a path of personal growth. You can do this, and you will. Just don't ever give up, turn your gray into sunshine as much as you can. God bless those who are currently fighting the fight.

I leave this to you, the one struggling with the breast pads they gave you because of breast cancer and losing your breasts, this is to you, the one with the colostomy bag who is constantly afraid to go out in public, this is for you, the current survivor, and loved ones who have lost their battle:

Father, help me keep my focus on you, when the pain, troubles, and hurt are overwhelming. Help me be faithful and good with blessings surrounding me. Please help my mind and soul be peaceful. Please strengthen my mind, body, and soul and heal me today. May the Holy Spirit Guide me in peace and comfort. Amen.

May God Bless you all and keep you safe.

Kali, xoxo

21

ARE YOU THERE GOD?

IT'S ME, LORI

BY LORI HERZOG

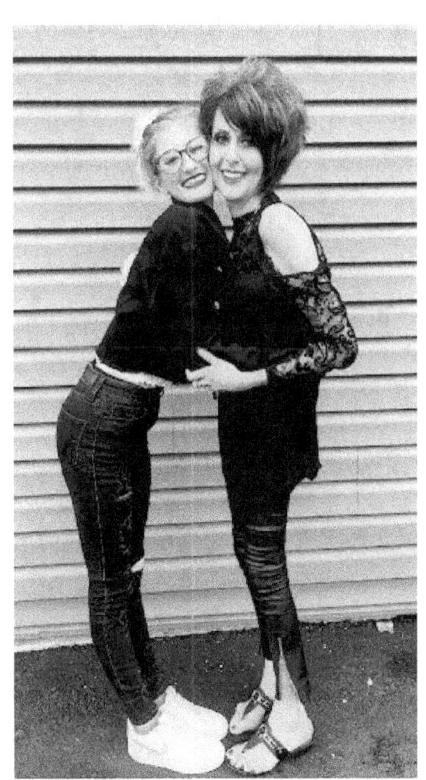

I grew up with the most loving mom there ever was. She was so confident and happy; my best friend. When I was 19 she discovered a small lump in her breast, but she didn't pursue medical care for it. I obviously realized later in life how oblivious I was to how serious this situation was. I walked daily, praying and thinking that this lump would just disappear; how wrong I was! I had just lost my grandmother shortly before this, so my mind didn't want to go there. My mother was my everything.

Let's fast forward 2 years…

I was 21 and she was 51. The lump was now the size of a chicken breast. I knew something had to be done. My mom worked at the Registration Desk at Elk County General Hospital. I began to make a plan to get her seen by a doctor because she refused to go to any for the past 10 years. I contacted two very close friends of hers that also worked at the hospital with her. They in turn got her an appointment with a surgeon; however, my mother was unaware of this. One of her friends came and wheeled her down in her desk chair to the doctor's office while the other one covered for her at the registration desk.

My worst fear came to pass. She was scheduled to have surgery within days of her appointment. She ended up having stage 4 breast cancer and had a mastectomy and lymph nodes removed. The cancer had spread.

My husband Dave and I had just built our home, so I insisted that she come to stay with us. She agreed and came to stay with us. It was heart-wrenching experience for me over a long period of time. Watching her go through chemo was hard; she lost her hair and was sick a lot. She was my mother and I loved her more than life itself.

She eventually became her old self again and all was well until seven years later when my worst fear came true. Her breast cancer had metastasized to every bone in her body. I had her to six different hospitals within two and a half months of her diagnosis.

In the meantime, my husband and I had been trying to conceive for two and half years with no success. I had a great gynecologist; he tried different procedures and fertility medications on me, I yearned to be able to tell my mother she was going to be a grandmother before she passed.

Exactly one week before she went to be with Jesus I found out I was pregnant. I was so excited to tell her. She was now a patient at the hospice unit in the hospital. But I got a chance to tell her that I was finally with child. She looked at me and gave me a thumbs up sign.

After my mother passed, I have never been the same. I miss her so very much. I wish she would have had a chance to meet her four beautiful granddaughters and two grandsons.

I knew I needed to be in tune with my body, it seemed that cancer ran in our family.

My mother died from breast cancer, my grandmother died from stomach cancer, my great grandmother died from colon cancer and her sister, my great Aunt had breast cancer. Therefore, I knew I needed to be very vigilant about my health care.

I began getting mammograms at the age of 30, and I made sure I went for my yearly PAP smear and checkup!

In 2017, I decided it was time for me to have genetic testing to see if any cancers might rear their ugly heads in the future. I tested positive for a gene mutation called CDH1.With that diagnosis I would eventually get breast cancer and stomach cancer at some point and potentially pass it on to my daughters. CDH1 is an extremely rare type of cancer, only 1% to 3% of world's population get it and it has a 15% five year cancer survival rate. This gene mutation was only discovered in 1998. This was two years after my mom had passed. I had a big decision to make.

I opted for a double mastectomy with reconstruction. Afterwards I was set up with Hahne Cancer Center and all the great doctors in Pittsburgh.

My breast cancer journey was nothing but pure hell.

I found out that I already had lobular breast cancer in my right breast. They found it during the biopsy. Thank God I had opted for the double mastectomy. My reconstruction journey didn't go as planned. I had a doctor that would NOT listen to me and let me suffer three and half months with cellulitis in my right breast. I was in the hospital more than I was home during this time. I had 2 tissue expanders and an implant that literally exploded in my chest.

A stranger found me passed out in the parking lot at my apartment house, picked me up and put me on the porch during a torrential rainstorm. Luckily, a friend passed by and saw me there and got me into my apartment. I was taken to the hospital and then transferred to Magee's Women's Hospital in Pittsburgh. I was septic and I almost died. I spent two weeks in the hospital there. I didn't know who I was and where I was. While I was in the ER an angel in disguise came up to me and said "I know why you are here and I think you need this." She handed me the business card for a woman plastic surgeon in Pittsburgh that is known as "The dream team."

From my first appointment, I knew I was in the best place possible. She worked her magic on me for a very long time. It took almost 2 years before I finally got my new breast. Her team did were amazing and I was so grateful to that woman who gave me her card. I had to go through several procedures and I always felt I was in the best hands possible. I placed my complete faith in her, I knew I was going to be okay.

I got a phone call from my gastroenterologist one day wanting to know if I was willing to talk to a lady who had just been diagnosed with the same mutation, CDH1. They said that I was the only one in the UPMC system with the same mutation. They explained she was having a really hard time with it and just wanted me to talk to her. They gave me her name and number; it's been six years and we still keep in touch. It still amazes me that I was the only one with that mutation that they had in the system.

Then it was Thanksgiving week, 2018. I had my second endoscope in Pittsburgh. It wasn't long before my doctor called me with more devastating news. I had stomach cancer and they wanted to do a complete gastrectomy on me. This would mean the removal of my entire stomach! I remember saying during Thanksgiving dinner, "This is going to be the last good meal I'll ever eat again."

The day came to get my surgery that included at least a two week stay in Shadyside Hospital, in Pittsburgh. After my surgery they tried a feeding tube which didn't work out so well, it made me deathly sick. My doctor started sending a variety of foods daily for me "pick at" to see what I could tolerate. When I went into the hospital, I weighed 158lbs and I was down to 88lbs at my lowest weight. In the weeks to months following my gastrectomy, it was a struggle to keep food down. I had severe heartburn and would throw up all the time. The acid from throwing up made my beautiful teeth turn brittle and fall out.

To this day, anytime I go anywhere I have to be aware of my surroundings. I never know when I will need a bathroom right away. I have lost a lot of control over my body. I still struggle with food, I am often asked "How do you eat without a stomach?" I have a tube connected from my esophagus to my small intestine. I have to be very careful of what I eat and how I eat. Small portions, nothing spicy, nothing too heavy, and no going back for seconds! I currently weigh 103 lbs and have maintained that weight for 3 years.

Having my stomach removed has caused me some other issues that I have had to learn to live with and take proper precautions for. I have hypoglycemia now, so I have to always make sure I have glucose tablets within reach for when these attacks come one. It is hard to know sometimes if I am eating enough or not, I am still trying to figure everything out.

What worries every parent is if we pass this gene on. I didn't want to pass it on to my four beautiful daughters! Three of them decided to get tested, and with such relief they were negative for the mutated gene. My fourth daughter wasn't quite ready.

My daughter Kali got pregnant and had our sweet little grandson Roman. After about a year, she came to me and decided it was time to get tested. Now that she was a mother, she wanted to do what was best for him.

That is when mine and Kali's lives would change forever. We are very close and very connected, more than ever. But that is her story to tell.

I live my life day by day, surrounded by weekly doctors' appointments. I get injections every three months to flush the estrogen out of my system since my cancer, like my mother's, was estrogen-fed. I have to make sure to get my monthly B-12 shots, blood work and take all my vitamins with all my medications. I don't travel very far anymore, maybe about 30 miles to the next town, mostly for doctors' appointments.

My life has changed drastically. I was always busy, up at the crack of dawn and ready to take on my day. I miss my old life before cancer. I sleep a lot and I have to nap a lot. I live with fear all the time. I have a beautiful family and I plan on sticking around as long as I can for my grandchildren and my pets. I have the sweetest fur babies in the world. They love me as much as I love them. My 2 beautiful cats and my sweet dog, Allie bring so much joy to my life.

What keeps me going? I have faith that has kept me strong through all of this.

22

FOREVER CHANGED

BY CHRISSY NUSSBAUM KEEBLER

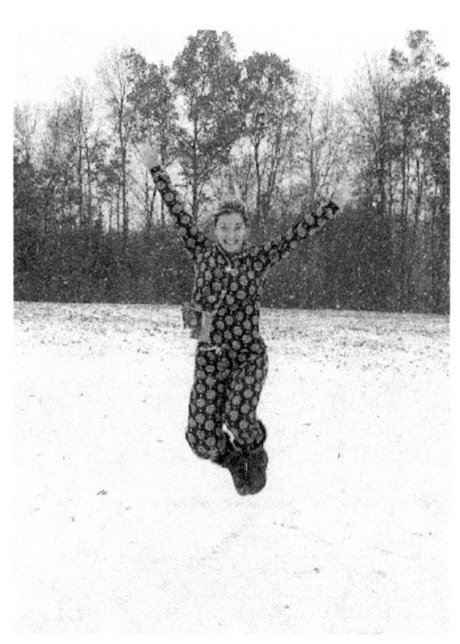

I t was the Saturday before Mother's Day in 2018. I was cooking breakfast for my family and brushed my flour-covered hands on my thighs as I typically do when I am cooking. I felt a lump in my upper thigh area, something I had not felt prior. It was a little smaller than the size of a golf ball. I instantly panicked, thinking the worst and asked my husband about it. He said it's probably just a swollen lymph node in response to a minor infection and to just keep an eye on it. Deep down in my heart, I knew it was cancer though. I waited about a week or two and called my family doctor. She initially was not too concerned and thought it was probably due to an infection and ordered bloodwork just in case. I was put on an antibiotic for a couple days to see if there was any response. In a few days, my doctor's office called me to give me the results of my bloodwork. My routine CBC was perfect, everything looked great! I still remember thinking great, no need to worry then, I'm fine! My doctor felt differently, since the lump was still there, she wanted to see me again to see if she noticed any change. Long story short, there was no change and she recommended that I get a biopsy to be safe. Due to insurance approvals, they required an ultrasound of the area prior to the biopsy. A few days later I had the ultrasound and shortly thereafter I got a call from my doctor's office with the report. The ultrasound showed metastasized cancer with lymph node involvement. My heart instantly sank. I was 39 years old, with 4 children, and 3 of them were little, ages 4,6, and 9. I called my husband at work, and I just remember him saying start making phone calls.

My family physician's office started by calling a local general surgeon that I knew and trusted. They could only see me for a consult at the end of July. I couldn't wait one month and a half, I would surely lose my mind during that time. They were going to call some Pittsburgh hospitals to see what they could do. I had an older friend who was on the board at Cleveland Clinic and always told me that if I ever needed anything medically to not hesitate to call him. As much as I didn't want to have to "use" him, I gave him a call because I was desperate. Don Fleming, God rest your soul, you were a saving grace to me. He made a phone call and told me that someone would be in contact with me very soon. I got a call from them shortly after and was scheduled for a few days to a week out with a general surgeon. She had told me that I was put on their cancelation list though should get something sooner. This was Monday, June 18th. We were to leave for a beach vacation the next day after work. That Tuesday morning around 10am, I got a call from the general surgeon's office in Cleveland. They would have a cancellation for 4pm that day if I could make it. I said yes! I called my mom to come babysit my younger kids and called my in-laws to see if they would drive me to Cleveland and off, we went. After a short visit with him, he scheduled me for a biopsy for the following Tuesday, June 26th. We knew there was nothing that we could do staying home, so we decided to leave for our vacation the next day to try to distract us.

Vacation was nice but it was hard. I kept thinking about the "what-ifs".

The 26th came and once again, I had my mom keep my little kids and my mother-in-law drove me to Cleveland. They took my blood pressure, and it was very high. They asked me if it was always this high and I responded no, I am a nervous wreck. They thought I was nervous for the procedure, but I was nervous for the results. The anesthesiologist came in and said that he was going to give me something to help me relax. He was great. He kept telling me that he understood what I was going through and asked me "where can I send you". I responded, "send me to the Caribbean"! We laughed and that was the last thing that I remembered until I woke up. They ended up taking the entire lymph node to make sure they had a good sample, so the incision was larger than I expected. The doctor told me that I would probably hear from him in 10 days, so I began the countdown.

Friday night the 29th I had a terrible toothache. The next morning, it was still killing me so I called my dentist and he got me right in. I got there and sure enough I had broken 2 teeth. One was repairable but one was not. He and I decided that I would call an oral surgeon on Monday to see about getting me in to get it pulled and get an implant put in, so he prescribed me antibiotics in the meantime, so it didn't get infected. Monday, July 2nd my mom had came over to swim with the kids since I wasn't allowed to swim yet with my incision. It was around 4pm and my phone rang. It was

Cleveland Clinic. I ran into the house to answer. I don't remember much from that phone call except hearing "you have Non-Hodgkins Lymphoma" and that it is something that I am going to have to learn to live with. I didn't know what all that meant at the time. I was crushed. I was scared. I instantly called my husband at work and gave him the news. He was in disbelief and didn't say too much. I then went out and told my mom the news. We both mentioned that this was the type of cancer that my aunt had a few years ago and that she had chemo and was doing well. We tried to keep that in our minds. I came back in the house and my husband called me back. The news set in and he stated that he was cancelling his patients for the rest of the day and coming home. I called my sister, and she was on her way over to my house to pick up my kids so my husband and I could process everything. My next phone call was to my Pastor asking for him to pray for me. Within 30-45 minutes of getting the call with my diagnosis, I got a call from a Medical Oncologist office from Cleveland Clinic to set up my appointment. The receptionist explained that I was going to need a PET scan, bloodwork, and a bone marrow biopsy to stage my cancer. A bone marrow biopsy? I don't want to have a bone marrow biopsy! I hate needles in my back, and I always heard how painful bone marrow biopsies were and now I had to face that. She scheduled these appointments and then for me to see the doctor in 2 weeks. I remember asking "2 weeks, is that really okay to wait that long?" She could sense my panic and told me that she was going to let me speak with the doctor himself. How many times does that happen? He got on the phone with me and fully explained the process. He told me that my cancer was "non-aggressive and very slow growing" so 2 weeks was perfectly fine to wait. He told me that if he felt I needed it sooner that he would make it happen, but he didn't see that need. He also explained to me that most times with my condition, radiation and watch and wait is usually the best treatment option. I had a hard time registering this, what does he mean watch and wait? However, even just that brief conversation, I trusted him. I knew he was the right doctor for me. That night while the kids were gone, led to lot of tears of just my husband and I sitting on the couch. I just kept going through the "what-if's". He kept setting me straight, even though I knew it was going through his mind too. He kept telling me, new treatments come out every day. Let's just focus on getting 5 years out. I'm tearing up just reliving all of this. This was the worst feeling of my life, by far. I have never been so scared. The next day I called my dentist back and gave him my news and told him that I just needed to get this tooth pulled because I had no idea what I was in for. I kept thinking, why is all of this happening at once? What is going on? I am telling you about my broken tooth because it will play a role in the future.

Over the next few weeks, I did tons of "research" aka Googling everything known to man about Non-Hodgkins Lymphoma. It stressed me out more and made things so much worse! So, to anyone out there reading this – DON'T

GOOGLE!! During this time, I got very depressed. I cried a lot! I felt as if I did something wrong. I had a very hard time facing people after getting this diagnosis. I had gone through a lot in my life already and never wanted to show weakness to anyone. I had my oldest daughter when I was just 16 years old and fought not to be a statistic. With the help of my parents and family, I finished high school, went to college, got a bachelor's degree in accounting, and held a great job as a Controller at our local car dealerships. But this, this had me at my worst. I just wanted to sit in a corner and cry. I wanted to avoid people. My friends and family pushed me to not let me do that of course. I ended up taking a leave from work. My husband and I had talked about me quitting my job many times due to our kids schedules and such, but I could never take that step. I worked hard to get to where I was, and I couldn't give up that independence…. until cancer hit. It hit me like a ton of bricks. I needed to be with my family right now. Suddenly work wasn't on the front burner. I almost felt like God was trying to push me in a different direction, but I wasn't listening and that He needed to push me harder. He needed to shake my world in only a way that he knew that I would respond. And I did.

My further testing and appointments came. I remember the night before my appointment to meet my oncologist, I got my PET scan results released to me through my online patient portal. I remember reading my report and thinking my cancer had spread to my bones and I really thought I was dying. I even packed a suitcase for my appointment because I was convinced that I was getting admitted and starting treatment asap. Another note – don't read your reports and try to interpret yourself! My interpretation could not have been further from the truth. On my way to Cleveland that morning, my mom had text me good luck and that she loved me. I remember telling her that I have never been so scared in all my life. I am sure looking back that broke her heart, but I was. Finally time to meet with the oncologist. He was a very straight forward almost intimidating doctor, but he was awesome. We knew we weren't getting any sugar-coated version of the truth; we were getting the actual truth. He explained to me that my PET scan showed lymphoma in my thigh. It had grown out from that original lymph node, but it was localized. That meant that it was not anywhere else in my body. That was a huge relief! Finally, some better news! He explained that Non-Hodgkins Lymphoma while not curable is very treatable. It will more than likely be something that I must deal with for the rest of my life, however, it would not affect my life expectancy unless it would turn to a more aggressive type. He instructed me to monitor myself for symptoms. Since my subtype was still up in the air, to watch for enlarged lymph nodes, night sweats, fevers, chills, etc. He stated that this can come back in my eyes, so to watch for any symptoms there as well. He explained what he thought my treatment plans would entail but we now needed to do the dreadful bone marrow biopsy. My husband was in with me holding my hand the whole time throughout the procedure. The doctor was talking about the recent firework displays and was asking if we watched any. He was trying hard to engage me in conversation to distract me, but I just wasn't having it. HAHA The biopsy didn't take very long, maybe 15-20 minutes if that. While it was uncomfortable, I think my mind made the process worse. At this time, my doctor explained the many different subtypes of Non-Hodkins Lymphoma and that my initial biopsy results were not 100% clear on my subtype, so he wanted some further testing done to be sure.

Lymphoma can hide in places. He wanted me to have a colonoscopy and an endoscopy done to verify that my GI Tract was free of lymphoma. He called one of our local GI doctors himself and explained the situation. They got me in very soon after. In recovery, the doctor explained to me that he did not see any signs of lymphoma, but he took samples and would send them away just to be sure. My husband and I celebrated this news a bit as things are going in the right direction now. Shortly after that, I received a call from Cleveland stating that my bone marrow biopsy was negative for lymphoma! I felt like the weight of the world was lifted! We then spoke about my treatment plan. I will say that cancer plays tricks on your mind, and you are always on guard. A week after my bone marrow biopsy, I noticed one morning as we were heading out of town that I had a hive on my back, right at my biopsy site. I instantly thought it was infected, I quickly messaged my doctor a picture of it and he really didn't think it looked like anything but he called me in a prescription just to be safe and ease my mind, I think. Well later that night, I realized that it wasn't even my biopsy site but about 2 inches away from it and it was more than likely a bug bite. My husband and I just laughed and laughed at our paranoia.

My treatment plan would consist of 15 radiation treatments to my left thigh and 4 weekly doses of Rituxan, which is a monoclonal antibody medication. I went and met with a radiation oncologist in Cleveland, and she was great. We loved her too. At one point, she could see the concern on my husband's face, and she looked at him and said, "she's going to be fine!" She then said "girl, there is no need for you to drive 8 hours a day for 15 minutes of treatment when someone local to you can do this". She went above and beyond. We told her about our local cancer center, and she personally called them and discussed what type of equipment they used. She verified that it was the same equipment that she would use, so she arranged a treatment plan with a more local cancer center. My medical oncologist in Cleveland did the exact same with my Rituxan treatments. He developed the treatment plan and my local center followed it and contacted him with any questions. I started the Rituxan treatments first since those appointments were available first. There is a risk of allergic reactions with Rituxan so the medication is given very slowly via an IV and you are monitored for any signs. These treatments would take about 6 hours per day. When I would first get there, I would get an IV, get bloodwork ran, get Tylenol, a Benadryl, and a steroid to combat any reaction. These treatments did not cause me many side effects. I would get headaches once they were finished, which could have come from the steroids too for all I know, and I would get very tired. The nurses at my local cancer center were absolutely amazing and joked and actually made it fun to be there. Don't get me wrong, it was tough to be in the treatment room and see all the people suffering from this terrible disease but also encouraging to see others fighting along with you. When you get diagnosed with cancer, no matter the type, you instantly have a connection with people. Complete strangers support you, encourage you, and are just there for you. It's definitely life changing. I completed those four treatments without any allergic reactions luckily and it was time for radiation. They did not want me to have both treatments at once, since it does weaken your immune system and for me it was not necessary.

The first appointment with radiation consisted of getting my "tattoos", which were five dots used to align the machine and getting my cast made. It's very important when getting radiation to be in the same position every time so the beam hits exactly where it is supposed to so they form a cast so to speak that my legs would lay in for each treatment so I wouldn't move. I really did not notice any side effects from this radiation, besides hair loss on my thigh which surprised me because at the time I didn't know that was a side effect of radiation. I finished my treatments and rang that bell!

Woohoo, I am done with treatments, I can get on with my life, right? Not quite. When I was actively going through treatments, I felt comfortable because I was fighting, I was doing everything that I could do for this disease. When I stopped, anxiety kicked in again. That depression kicked in again. The questions started… did the treatments work? Will it come back? When will it come back? What treatments will I have to endure next time? Will it be more aggressive next time? Too many questions and no answers for them. This is when I thought it was time to talk to a counselor. I needed additional help to get through this next stage. My counselor gave me a post it note with "you can't grow in comfort" written on it. I can't tell you how many messages God gave me over the next several months that always revolved around getting out of my comfort zone. He used the counselor to set that thought in motion.

I turned to my faith like I never have before. I grew up going to a Catholic school, going to church with my family every Sunday, and even multiple times a week during school but I needed more. God is what I needed to help me get through this next phase. I never really knew the Bible. One day during this whole diagnosis, I remember having a bad day. I was crying non-stop, trying to hide my tears from my little kids because we only told them very little details. The 3 were too little to understand fully and I did not want them worrying. It's bad enough my oldest daughter had to endure this. Anyways, I just remember being in my bedroom and being completely empty and dropping to my knees and asking God for help. Asking him to guide me, give me direction, because I can't do this on my own. In looking back now, I wish I would have written everything down because I thought I would remember all the details on the signs He gave me throughout my journey, but I don't. He opened my eyes like they were never opened before. I would see signs everywhere telling me that things were going to be okay. I joined a Bible Study at our church and would open up with these girls and how I came to the realization that getting cancer was actually one of the best things that ever happened to me. Figure that one out, I know! I needed to be at my weakest in order to grow both in my faith and personally. And wow did God show me things that I always overlooked before. It ended up becoming a joke with one of my closest Bible Study friends "Yeah, I am sure that was just a coincidence"! It was an amazing feeling.

A few months after finishing up my treatments, I was scheduled for another PET scan to make sure things were looking good. I got a call on November 15, 2018, from my Oncologist that my scan was clear, no cancer! This was the best news! We were in the middle of a snowstorm, and I remember telling my husband who happened to be off work that morning that I was going out in the snow and dancing in my pajamas! And so, I did! He captured a photo of it, and it is my most favorite picture ever! I shared it on Facebook that day and on every November 15th from that day on, well until 2023 that is. I immediately called my oldest daughter and the rest of my family to share the news! Our younger 3 got an early dismissal so my husband and I were able to share the news with them as well! Following was a celebration dinner with my oldest daughter, Kayla, and some of our close friends who stood by our side the past five months helping us to get through this. I can not thank them enough for always being right there to come hang out with us at a moment's notice.

I met with my Cleveland doctor shortly after and he recommended maintenance Rituxan for 2 years following my remission to help keep me in remission longer. He had warned me prior that we might do maintenance, so I knew this was a possibility. I would receive a Rituxan treatment every other month for 2 years. I walked out of his office in tears because I just didn't want to have to think about this anymore (more than what is always in the back of my mind). I knew it was a good thing to do but I was still disappointed. However, I put my big girl pants on and did what I needed to do. In January of 2019, I officially resigned from my Controller position and became a full time stay at home Mom and volunteer. I just knew God was telling me that it was time for a change, so I listened this time. It was hard. I had liked my job. I held that job for 19 years. I just couldn't mentally go back.

I continued volunteering at my kids' school and at our church. I continued with my maintenance treatments without any reactions. I had follow-up visits with my local oncologist and routine bloodwork, and everything continued to be good. On one of my trips home from my checkup, God gave me a clear indication that I was to run for our local School Board Director position that was opening up. It was something that I had thought about in the prior years but never acted on but now it was clear that I needed to do this. So, I ran for the position and was elected. It is very weird in the directions God takes you when you stop and listen. I ended my maintenance treatments in November of 2020 amid the Covid pandemic. I was extremely nervous during the pandemic because I knew my immune system was weakened with my treatments, so I was very cautious. I was lucky to not have contracted the virus while I was receiving them.

I had a follow up PET scan in December of 2020 and all was still clear! This time, my Cleveland oncologist did not see a need for future PET scans or CT scans unless I was having symptoms because the radiation associated with them could cause me more harm than good with my type of cancer. So, I just need to be aware of my symptoms and watch for lumps, bumps, etc. He stated that new studies have shown that radiation may be potentially curative, and I was so thrilled to hear this! I was now on annual checkups with him and every 6 months checkups with my local oncologist. Since my diagnosis I try to reach out to anyone that I know that is facing this disease, especially those younger and with kids. I did not know of anyone when I was facing this and I really wish that I had.

Since 2020 I have been feeling great and life has been going great. Still a bit of PTSD would appear out of nowhere somedays, like the time I broke another tooth. When that happened, my diagnosis flooded my brain and had me in a panic. The last time I broke a tooth, I had just received my diagnosis. Now, the broken tooth and the cancer had no correlation but in my mind that's what I could recall. I talked myself down on that one and realized that little triggers would continue and vowed to try my best to work through them as best as possible.

I now have 2 grandbabies, one boy and one girl, this is something that I prayed for during my cancer battle that I would get to see. My little kids were all in school now and I was feeling the need to get out of the house and be productive. I am still the President of the PTO at my son's school, still on the School Board, volunteer at our church, I picked up a small Secretary/Accounting position at our church and was looking to start my own independent accounting office. My kids' schedules became more demanding as they are getting older and joining more after school activities. I didn't have time for my Bible Studies, etc. like I did before. Just when things started picking up with that, some personnel changes happened at my husband's chiropractic office, and we decided it was best for me to step into the Office Manager position there. I dove into learning this job and trying to help him grow his practice. I became very busy, very fast with trying to juggle all the roles that I took on in just a very short period of time. My husband who had been trying to hire an associate chiropractor for years, finally found a promising one. We were busy working on the details and contracts for months making sure everything was perfect.

One night during late July / August of 2023 I noticed a weird discoloration in my right eye and thought I must have broken a blood vessel or something. I didn't think much of it at the time. After a few weeks or two of watching it, I showed it to my husband. He thought the same thing, weird you must have done something to it. Then it hit me. Cleveland told me to watch my eyes! Could this be what he meant? At this point, I knew again, it was back. Although I worry about everything, I am always paranoid that something is cancer, but I think all cancer survivors have those feelings. I told my husband what I was thinking. Deep down, I think he knew too but he told me "You always think everything is cancer, you need to stop worrying so much". We went back and forth on this for a little bit that night. Monday morning came and he said to me "call the eye doctor and go get it checked out". When he says it's time to go to the doctor, you know he's concerned. So, I started panicking again.

I explained my concerns to my local eye doctor, and she got me right in. She was dumbfounded. She had never seen anything like this before either. She stated that overall, my actual eye looked great, but the discoloration and puffiness in my conjunctiva looked concerning. She referred me to a surgeon and said that if she had to give it a diagnosis, she would say it appears to be some type of tumor. The surgeon could see me relatively soon, but I knew I needed to start calling "my people". I called my local oncologist, and they were not aware of lymphoma coming back in the eye and they instructed me to see the local eye doctor. I wasn't settling for this; I knew I had to get to somewhere with experience of lymphoma in the eye to rule it out. Then I reached out to my Cleveland Oncologist through my patient portal and explained what I was seeing and sent him a picture. As I was pulling into the surgeon's office for my appointment, the Cleveland office called me and said that they wanted me to see their Ocular Oncologist. I ended up keeping the appointment and again this doctor knew it was something but wasn't sure what it was. She could feel the mass and said I should follow up with Cleveland. I have found out that Ocular Oncologists are very rare and so therefore they are extremely busy! I had to wait a few weeks to get in to see him, but it was well worth the wait.

When the day finally came to see the Ocular Oncologist, he walked into the exam room and right away spotted symptoms that I had never seen. He told me that this was in fact lymphoma, not in the actual eye itself, but in the orbit of my eye. He stated that it was pushing my eye up and out. The slight discoloration and little bit of mass that I could see was just because it was getting pushed up enough for me to see it to notice it was there. He diagnosed me before any imaging or biopsies. I was crushed to say the least. I figured that my cancer was back, but it didn't matter none the less. He could sense my anxiety and told me about 10 times, "this is 100%

treatable with radiation, you are going to be fine". He has seen many of these, and I was his second one that morning. After my appointment, he did slit lamp photos of my eye to get a better idea on the size of the mass and scheduled me for a biopsy. A biopsy of your eye sounds fun, doesn't it?! My husband and I walked back to our car, and I made it to the car and I just lost it. I cried an ugly cry and just when I thought I was stopping, I cried some more. I honestly felt with all my heart, that I was cured, that it was gone for good. I didn't have the heart to tell everyone yet, so I waited for the official results once I got the biopsy.

On October 30th, 2023, my sister drove me to Cleveland for my biopsy. I ended up with 8 stiches in the conjunctiva of my eye and a nice eye patch just in time for Halloween. It wasn't very painful. It was very scratchy, irritated, and just gave you a headache in that eye. I ended up getting a very nice black eye that lasted for a few weeks. I got questioned a few times about who punched me and had one guy that was ready to either call the cops or punch my husband in the face, I'm not sure which one! We clarified what had happened and we all laughed. I thanked him for having my back though! During the time I was waiting for my results, I received a CT scan to look for more. It was clear! What a huge relief!

During this time, I had a hard time connecting with God. I knew he healed me before and I kept praying but it was different this time around, it was hard. I felt angry, let down, abandoned, but I also felt that since I have been so busy with life and neglected my relationship with Him that if I turn to Him now, that it looks like "oh so now I am good enough because you need me". Cancer is tough. It gives you all kinds of crazy emotions and I can't even explain them all. Or then again, maybe it's just me! I again reached out to my Bible Study friend who is my rock when it comes to stuff like this and explained to her how I was feeling. Once again, she was right there for me to let me know what that is not God talking to me but the evil one trying to push me further away from God. That put things back into perspective for me.

I had to wait 18 days for my next appointment to find out the biopsy results. Yes, I already knew what it was, but boy did I hope it wasn't lymphoma again. My husband and I went to that appointment that day and we had a 3.5 hour wait to see the doctor. They prepare you that it could be up to a 4 hour wait but it seemed like we sat there for a month that day! We finally got called in and he reported that it was in fact my lymphoma again. The good news was that it had not changed types. He looked at me again and said, "I told you, 100%.... not 99, 98, 96, or 92%....100%. As much as I trust these doctors, it's still hard not to question, "how do you know?', "what if it doesn't go as planned?" Let's face it… he doesn't know that God's plans are for me! He went on to tell me that treatment would consist of 12-15 radiation treatments to that eye, but since eye lymphoma is so rare, he wanted me to go to "his" guy. His radiation oncologist treated his last 250 patients and that he kills it 100% of the time. I couldn't argue with that, I wanted the best. I knew this was going to be hard on my family since we live 3.5 hours away from Cleveland, in good weather.

As I said prior, I had many obligations, and they were on the forefront of my mind. Who is going to help my husband with the kids, laundry, dinners, and keeping up the house? I am President of the PTO and in just a few weeks, I was chairing a huge Breakfast with Santa event. How could I possibly pull his event off if I may or may not even be in town? I was trying and trying to figure out how I was going to make this all work for everyone and not let anyone down. Notice, I said how "I" was going to pull this all off. Like most women I know, I'm too proud to ask for help. Pride is not a good thing to have. I always think that I can work harder and accomplish it all. As the news traveled about my diagnosis, the outreach of support was overwhelming. I had people offering to take my kids when they were off school, do my laundry, cook them dinners, and run them anywhere they needed to go. My wonderful group of PTO girls all stepped up and divided up the tasks for our Breakfast with Santa so I did not have to worry about a thing. And the event was fantastic! I learned a valuable lesson from God during this time around, it's okay to ask for and accept help. We can not do everything on our own. Once again, God overwhelmed me with emotion as I sat there soaking up the lesson that God taught me through this battle.

The radiation oncologist scheduled me for a consultation for the next week. Once again, my sister and I headed out to Cleveland the day after Thanksgiving to meet with him. When he came into the exam room, he was very informative. He made sure to tell me that my cancer is not like other types of cancer. He went on to say that my type of Non-Hodgkins Lymphoma will continue to do this the rest of my life and it's just an "inconvenience". He explained that this diagnosis will not affect my God given life span unless my type was to change to an aggressive type, which is a 5% chance for me. He again told me; this is 100% treatable with radiation. This was the 3rd doctor to tell me this. I must trust them. So, every time I would start worrying and thinking the worst, I would reset myself and say 100% treatable. He was great. He explained the process, the side effects, everything. He told me that I would experience a sunburn on my face around that eye, a dry eye that waters constantly, I would lose my eyelashes, but he was going to try his best to save my eyebrows. Yes, to those reading this that don't know, radiation does cause hair loss too. He explained that I would have to come back for CT scans because he wanted to try his best to avoid my retina, optic nerve, etc. if at all possible, to avoid any vision complications. I was also informed that there is a chance of me developing a cataract within 3 years of receiving radiation to my eye, but it would be easily taken care of if that should happen. He also explained that I would get a mask made during those tests as well that I would have to wear during treatments and that this mask gets clipped to the table to keep you from moving.

A few weeks later, the authorization to proceed was received from my insurance company and I went back out to get my CT scans and my mask made. For those wondering, the mask consists of warm, mesh, plastic sheet that is laid across your head and they proceed to start shaping it to your face before it cools. Once they are happy with the shape, I had to lay there for about 10-15 minutes and let it cool and take shape. Once it was ready, it was hardened and shaped to my face/head.

I knew we were getting close to the holidays and was really hoping that I would get to start treatment right away and be done before Christmas but that didn't happen. I received the notice that I was going to start radiation on Monday, December 18, the week before Christmas. I was so sad at this point. Christmas is my favorite time of year, and I didn't want to be away from home during Christmas, but God had other plans, I guess. I had searched out different options available to cancer patients on lodging and was prepared to go myself during the week and then come home on the weekends so my family could be available to help with my kids at home. My sister had other plans though. She insisted that I was not going out there by myself and that she was going with me. Her kids are grown and have houses of their own, so she said it was like a mini vacation to her. I fought her tooth and nail! I'm fine, I'm tough, I can do this myself! I didn't win the fight! Haha Friday, December 15, late afternoon, I get a call from Cleveland saying that they had to postpone my treatment start date until Tuesday the 19th. My heart sank, I questioned the poor nurse that called me on why. She stated that the machine that I was scheduled for had gone down that day and they did not get to run the proper safety protocols that they had to run for my setup, and they were not comfortable proceeding until they could do so. I completely understood and agreed that I wanted everything to be perfect, but I was annoyed to say the least. Now, my oldest son was at a wrestling tournament that day an hour and 45 minutes away. We were planning on heading to the tournament as soon as we got out of work to watch him for the weekend. About a half hour after my call from Cleveland, a parent at the wrestling tournament video chatted with us because my son was about to wrestle and that way, we could watch him. Well, he ended up breaking his leg during that match. We took him to the ER that night, but we needed to follow up with an orthopedic Monday, the day that I was supposed to start my treatments. I was like, Okay God, I see why I needed to get postponed. I was able to get him all taken care of and left early Tuesday for Cleveland for the week! It's funny how things work out!

Treatment was quick and easy that day. It took them longer to put my mask on and snap me to the table than for the actual 16 second treatment. The staff for my machine was awesome. Very caring individuals and made me feel comfortable right from the start. They gave me my schedule and went about and beyond to rearrange my treatment time for the day after Christmas and the day after New Year's Day so I would not have to leave to come back out on the holidays but rather leave early that morning for treatments. Not only was I able to be home with my kids longer, but it also saved me some money on hotel charges too. Our hotel offered free dinners and 3 free alcoholic drinks per night for each registered guest (over 21 for drinks) so we took advantage of that that night. We then settled into our hotel room for the night watching Christmas movies. It was time for bed, and I was in my bed and my sister was in her bed. We turned the lights off and my sister made a comment about how dark the room was except for the red lights on the TV. I said, "there is no red light on the tv". She said "yes, there is". I responded again, "no, there isn't." At this point she jumped up out of bed and went to the tv and said, "you mean that you can't see this red light?" From my position in bed, I could not see any red light. I sat up then and then I could see the red light. There was a little tent no smoking sign right in front of the red light, so from my bed you couldn't see it but from her bed you could. She said, "I was about ready to load you in the car and take you to the ER, I thought the treatment affected your vision! We laughed so hard at this and her panic and joked about it for the next 3 weeks. Just thinking about it again has me sitting here laughing!

Over the next three weeks, we did some shopping to get ready for Christmas, we went out to eat, went to see a movie, just relaxed in our hotel room. Some days, I would get this overwhelming exhaustion come over me, especially in my legs, and I would wind up in bed by 6-7pm for the night. I had to listen to my body and rest when I needed to and not try to push myself through it like I have always done before. Don't tell her, but I am glad she decided to go and hang out with me. I probably would have been a depressed mess for 3 weeks by myself. Every day when I arrived at the center, I would have to valet my car. There were 2 older valet guys at the cancer clinic that became my buddies. They would always tell me "I'll take good care of you; I have your back." They would always be a bright start to my day.

One thing that changed me when I was first diagnosed with cancer was my punctuality. I was always one of those people who was running late until I had any cancer related appointments. Now, I'm sometimes 1 hour early to places. I'm telling you, it's funny what all cancer does to you! So, I spent some time sitting in the waiting room waiting for the treatment because I was always so early. Some days, I would sit quietly, some days I would chat with spouses waiting while their significant others were getting treatments, some days I would be brought to tears at seeing the little ones leaving from their treatments.

One of my encounters remains very clear in my mind though. He was an older gentleman and very willing to talk. We talked about many different things, and we course talked about our diagnosis. He had what seemed to be an aggressive form of prostate cancer as he was receiving like 45 doses of radiation. He was on his 3rd last day when we first met, just like I was. He stated that you just have to trust in the Lord because that's the only thing that we can control in all of this. I told him that he was absolutely right! He looked at me very seriously and said, "are you a Christian?' I responded with "yes, I am". He told me how excited he was to hear that and showed me his Bible in his shirt pocket that he carries with him wherever he goes. At that moment, you could feel the bond that we formed. We talked for a few more minutes and he got called back for his treatment. I was still sitting there when he was done, and he came back over to talk to me. He told me how glad he was to have met me and that he would be praying for me every day. I then got called back so our conversation ended. When I got back out to the waiting room, I told my sister all about him. He really touched me that day. The strength, compassion, and support that you get from fellow cancer fighters and survivors is unlike anything else. You instantly have a bond with someone you know nothing about.

The next morning, I had an early treatment. When I arrived at valet, I have never seen it so busy. I waited in line to park for almost 15 minutes. By the time I checked in, I was not as early as I like to be, but as I walked into the main entrance, he was standing there. The older gentleman from the day before also had an early treatment that morning and was standing in the entrance waiting for his car. He looked at me to see if I would recognize him. I instantly did! His face got a huge smile on it. I stopped for a minute or two to check on him and see how he was doing and to make sure his treatment went well that morning. We both said, "1 MORE"! He again told me that he will be praying, and I said I would continue to do the same and I had to leave for my treatment. I was really hoping that I would see him the next morning so we could celebrate our end of treatments together, but unfortunately, I didn't. I don't know this man's name, but he is certainly not a stranger to me. God sent him to me or maybe I to him, I'm not sure, all I know is that he reaffirmed that we need to fight and trust in the Lord.

Treatments left me with some reminders of what I have been through. The fatigue lingered for a few weeks. Some days were worse than others, but this time around, I let myself nap because I knew I needed this to continue with my fight. I was sunburned as they called it. I had a pretty big circle ranging from mid-cheek, to above my eyebrow of redness. The worst of it came the week after I finished my treatments. It got to the point that it was purple from the burns. It was very dry, burned, and very sore to the touch. My eyeball itself was very sensitive, red, inflamed, and would get very tired especially after looking at computer screens, etc. for a few hours during the day. It would end up leaving me with a headache in that eye. I just realized that as I am finishing writing my story, that it is February 4th. My last treatment was exactly 1 month ago today. I am sure that is just another one of God's "coincidences" for me! Anyways, I still have some redness on my eye, still sensitive, and it waters like crazy but all in all I can't complain. I will follow up with my ocular and radiation oncologist in April for a check up to make sure there are no effects on my vision. I have a follow up with my medical oncologist at the end of June for a PET scan to make sure all is clear. Those tests are always nerve racking but they are a necessary evil that we cancer warriors must face.

Hopefully you are still reading with me here. My advice to everyone. Know your body! If you have a concern, don't dismiss it. You may not want to hear the answer, but you need to hear it. Be persistent in your care. Remember the old saying that the squeaky wheel gets the grease? Be the squeaky wheel! You only get one chance at this thing called life so fight and fight hard. Never give up. As for me, there is a good chance that my lymphoma will keep being an inconvenience throughout my life so as my husband says, I'm going to keep on grinding. I am going to own this cancer; it's not going to own me!

BEEN THERE, DONE THAT!

BY BETH PIFER

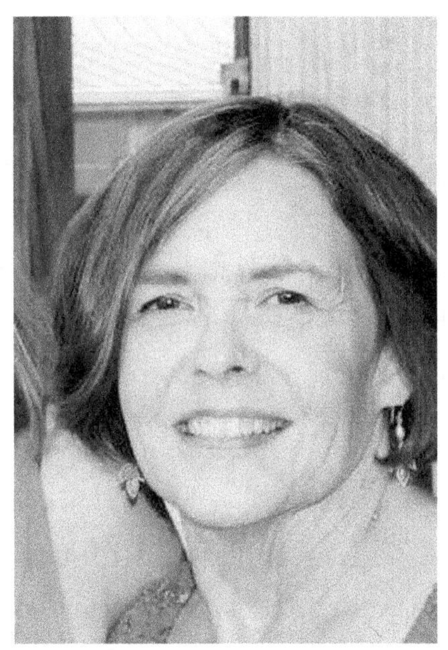

This has been a slogan of mine for years; "Been there, done that." Often I will follow that saying with, "and no, I didn't write a book." But now here I am, as Patty has asked me to write the book. Well, not the whole book, but here is my chapter.

My name is Beth Pifer. I am originally from Ridgway, PA, and now live in Grand Junction, CO. I graduated high school with Patty and many others who are contributing to this book. I struggled to think why anyone would want to read about my cancer journey. I guess there are things that I do want the reader to know if they are in the battle right now, or if they have a loved one who is fighting. You need to know that you are not alone, God is with you, and there is great power in prayer.

I was first exposed to the word cancer when I was a small girl. My grandfather "Grandpap Sue" had throat cancer. No one really seemed to know much about cancer back then. He had his own plate and silverware and slept in his own room. His eating utensils were washed separately from the rest of the dishes to ensure no one else "caught it" from him.

Next, there was my sweet Kalea, who I babysat. She was only an infant when she was diagnosed with brain cancer. I was babysitting her the night they ended up taking her to the hospital and air flighting her to Children's Hospital. After years of surgeries, treatments and struggles, she went to be with the Lord at age eight. I learned a great lesson from this little girl. That being, cancer is a personal struggle, and it is up to the individual to choose their own path. At a tender young age, she made the decision that there would be no more treatments, and heaven was the better alternative for her.

I joined the club that nobody wants to join in September of 2016. It was just one noticeable lump, but I already knew in my heart what it was. I had been feeling different for a long time. It started with the removal of the lump, the biopsy, meeting with the surgeon, choosing an oncologist, and making a plan. My prayer during this time was mainly to be guided to the right person to trust. It was imperative to me to have someone to trust at this point, and I chose Dr King.

My initial diagnosis wasn't bad, Follicular Lymphoma. But soon after, the PET scan revealed it was Stage 4. All things considered, this diagnosis was still not terrifying because according to my team, this was a slow growing cancer that would not require any treatment for up to ten years. Friends and family spent time checking WEBMD and Google for alternative outcomes. I held hope for a complete recovery for that ten years, but luck was not on my side.

According to what I was told, there is a small percentage of people with Follicular Lymphoma that have it morph into something else. In my case, it was back in less than a year with a vengeance, and it developed into Large Diffused B

Cell Lymphoma. Upon that diagnosis it took less than 72 hours to go from that doctor's appointment, to biopsy, to having a port placed, and to having my first of many, many chemotherapy treatments. The therapy was called RCHOP. This combination contains the chemotherapy drugs cyclophosphamide, doxorubicin hydrochloride (hydroxy-daunomycin), and vincristine sulfate (Oncovin), the targeted therapy drug rituximab, and the steroid hormone pred-nisone. Quite a cocktail!

My cousin Connie, who has the same cancer, came to stay for about 10 weeks. I probably didn't need the help but my husband Randy, needed to have someone with me while he worked, more so for his own peace of mind. I was able to keep working part-time for many months, However as the chemicals built up in my system, my mind became less sharp. As an accountant who is responsible for others' money, it is best to be in your sharpest mind. So that ended my career.

The thing I recall most during that time was the number of cures for cancer that people offered. I could not possibly try even half of them. I loved all the people that tried so hard to take this from me, however I just thanked them, took their information, but instead continued to trust God, and trust Dr King.

I did reach a point where I was considered to be in remis-sion. During that time, I decided to try an alternative treat-ment plan at the recommendation of my lovely friend Kelly, who is alive today as a result of Ozone treatments. The person leading this plan suggested some life changes from a book called, "Anti-cancer Living." So, armed with my book and my very own ozone machine, I marched forward into my new, healthy life. I was feeling better than I had in years!

Continuing to follow the recommendation of Dr King, I followed through with my yearly PET scan which, unfortunately revealed a wider spread of cancer cells than ever before. Cancer is a tricky one, and can't be trusted to stay gone, even when that is all we hope for. I had missed a clinical trial for the latest and greatest treatment at the time. So, according to my doctor, my option was more chemotherapy and the addition of a STEM cell transplant.

I could have gone many places, and done many other things, but I did not want to leave home. I began my treatments and was to have my STEM cells harvested, revamped, and replaced in Salt Lake City, UT. Keeping in mind my desire to stay home, I felt okay about this plan knowing that my husband Randy would simply relocate with me to Utah for the time. As the planning continued, nothing in the original blueprint went as planned. My body did not tolerate the new chemotherapy treatments. What was originally meant to take twelve weeks, took five and half months. The process of the STEM cell harvest was tedious yet interesting, to say the least, as I sat in a chair watching every drop of blood in my body leave and come back, six and half times.

After more rounds of chemo, I was at last off to Salt Lake to get my STEM cell replacement. We had hoped that Randy could join me and move with me during this harrowing experience. However, there was no option for Randy to join me, because it was then March of 2020, the height of COVID. Our family was crushed as now I was literally dropped off at the front door, no visitors allowed in the building and could only come back later and pick me up. You could not pay me enough to re-live this part of my life. I was a rock star though. With much prayer and some morphine, I was released in a record two and half weeks.

There have been ups and downs since that time. Some great days and some pain. Some radiation and some traveling. Some laughter and some tears. Some friends who have died of cancer and some who are living happily ever after. So what would I want you to know should you walk this road someday? I would want you to know that you are not alone. God has promised that He will never leave you or forsake you. If you end up in an isolation ward during a pandemic, you are not alone. I know this to be true. I was there, and the loving arms of my Lord Jesus Christ held me the whole time.

Now a little advice to those of you who love a person with cancer. "Let me know what I can do to help," just isn't enough. In the throes of treatment nobody knows what they need. Or perhaps it is more than can be articulated. Instead try, "I am at the ice cream shop, what is your favorite flavor?" Or, "Heads up, I am coming to vacuum and dust on Tuesday."

Try a variation of, "my famous lasagna is arriving on Friday." Or my dream scenario, "My window cleaner is coming to your house, pick a day, my treat!" You know the person you love better than they might know what they need during the battle with cancer. Take the initiative to be with, serve, and affirm them in this time. You may need to give more than they need to receive.

I will wrap up by sharing an illustration I have loved for many years of my life. Within the Winnie the Pooh clan there is Eeyore. Even though that sweet, sad donkey is basically clinically depressed, he still gets invited to participate in adventures and shenanigans with his friends. They never expect him to pretend to feel happy, they never leave him behind or ask him to change. They just show him love. Please, stay near to your afflicted friends and don't ask them to change the way they have decided to wield their sword for their own fight.

I am blessed and I am lucky. My husband is a great cheer-leader and loves me unconditionally. Our children live very close and have done whatever is asked of them to help. I have more friends than I can count; they came in and cleaned every corner of my house, which was a prerequisite for coming home after my transplant.

God has promised to lead us down every path in our lives and show us what path to take. For me, James 3:17 was very helpful with this. "But the wisdom that comes from heaven is first of all pure, then peace-loving, considerate, submissive, full of mercy and good fruit, impartial and sincere." I have based my cancer journey decisions on this scripture, and it has not failed me. God wants none to suffer, but to come to a saving grace.

Will I live a good long time, or will cancer take me? "To live is Christ and to die is gain" Philippians 1:21

IT IS WELL WITH MY SOUL

BY JACKI WOLFGANG SIMANIC

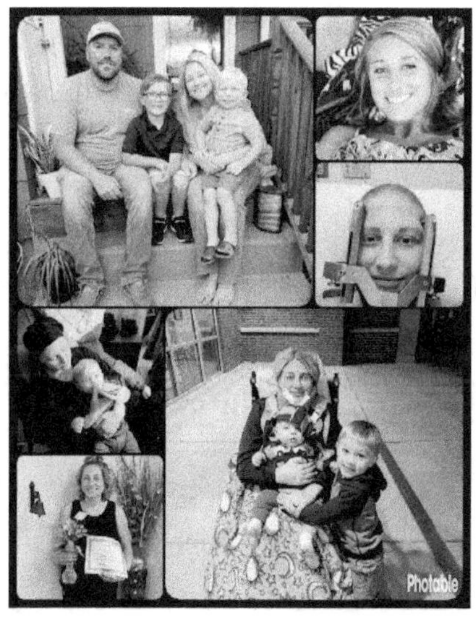

September 30, 2020 will forever be etched in my memory. It was the most devastating day that I was told I had Stage four HER2+ breast cancer. The word "cancer" altered my life in unexpected ways. It reshaped my perspective on what truly matters. It strengthened my relationship with God.

I was a 30-year-old newlywed who recently married my better half, Paul. We had a three-year-old son, a three-month old son, and a third child on the way. We were so excited for our growing family.

Shortly after I gave birth to our second son, I started experiencing back and hip pain. At first I brushed it off thinking it was symptoms of afterbirth. However, as the days went by the pain became unbearable. I made a chiropractor appointment thinking that would help relieve some pressure. That appointment was the best and worst decision of my life. If it wasn't for this appointment, I would not have known about my cancer.

After attending a couple of chiropractic sessions, my pain kept growing. I could hardly walk. The muscle spasms in my back were unreal. I laid on the couch screaming out in pain, wanting to die to take the agony away.

The next day, I went to the ER. Since I was expecting, I was unable to have any tests performed on me. The doctors opted for an x-ray. This showed the beginning of my problem, which was a break in my T4 and T5 area. I then had to have an MRI. My MRI appointment at my local hospital was scheduled for weeks away. I was in so much pain that my uncle drove me to an ER an hour and half away, to see if they could help more quickly. They would not give me an MRI. I finally got into a hospital twenty miles from home that had a cancellation. After I had the MRI, I was told I would need surgery. I had no idea how this was going to happen since I was expecting.

On September 29, 2020, my mom and I were on our way to see a back surgeon, 60 miles away, to discuss my options. Halfway there, I received a call from the back surgeon's office telling us to turn around. They reviewed my MRI and said they couldn't help me because I had something growing on my spine. I called my primary care physician to ask what I should do, and I was sent to neurology immediately. I was terrified, anxious, and nervous, however I knew my faith was bigger than my fear.

When I arrived at neurology, I was told I was way too young to have this kind of a back break. I was sent for a breast ultrasound which came back clear. I was then admitted to the hospital to do more testing. I was so scared and had no idea on the journey I was about to embark on. The doctor ruled out lymphoma and leukemia, and I was thankful it was neither of those. The doctors revisited my previous MRI and noticed white spots on my right pelvic bone. I was sent for a biopsy, and the results showed it was breast cancer.

I was shocked because I was told my breast ultrasound was clear. I was devastated as I hugged Paul tight and cried on his shoulder. I called my family and told them the news. As a family, we agreed for me to go to Cleveland Clinic in Cleveland, OH for the best care. I was then discharged from my local hospital. I went home to say goodbye to my family before traveling to the clinic. Our children were able to stay with my parents. Paul and I arrived in Cleveland later that night. Due to covid restrictions, Paul was not allowed to stay with me at night, only during the day. Once I was admitted, he had to stay in a hotel. We were upset and frustrated, however we knew I was in the best care. Who would have predicted that I'd be lying in a hospital bed alone, not knowing what I was going to face.

The next day, they had a mammogram for me. This showed I had two tumors in each breast. I could not believe what they just told me. They then took a biopsy of one to determine the type of cancer. It was stage four HER2+. All I could do was cry and think about my children. I was not afraid to die, however the thought of leaving my children was devastating. As this went on, I had a team of 17 doctors that discussed my case and made decisions together. Since the cancer was growing on my spine, the neurosurgeon did not want to do surgery on me because my case was too risky. The break was lying on my spinal cord, so I could have easily been paralyzed if I fell or hit the wrong spot. The break eventually ended up healing on its own, which is a miracle in itself.

My oncologist came up with a chemo plan. Since I was pregnant, my local cancer center would not accept me. We found a cancer center sixty miles from home that accepted me. I was discharged from Cleveland. Paul and I went to the cancer clinic for a consultation where they did blood work and learned my case. On our way home, I received a phone call from them, telling me to go to the nearest emergency room because I had fatal calcium levels.

I was admitted to my local hospital where the doctor told me my high calcium levels were caused by my pregnancy. I was told I or the baby would not make it through the nine months. My heart was shattered, and I didn't want to accept it. I was then taken back to Cleveland by ambulance.

When I arrived in Cleveland, I was told the same thing; neither the baby nor I would survive the pregnancy. I could not easily give up on the precious gift from God that He blessed me with. I rejected chemo. My doctors told me that without the medication, I would die. After talking with my family and the hospital's pastor, Paul and I made the decision for me to start chemo. I lost the baby. God showed me peace and comfort knowing I will meet her in heaven someday.

The next morning, I had a PET scan of my whole body. I had two tumors in each breast, on my liver and all of my bones. I lost five inches in height from compression fractures. After being bedridden for one month, I was ready to start my first chemo. I received it in my hospital bed and experienced the worst side effects such as chills and pain. I started losing my hair right away. Each day I would pull chunks of my hair out to the point that my sister had to shave my head. This was one of the most difficult physical appearances I had to accept as I always had long, thick blonde hair that girls would envy.

I struggled to achieve my same look as I was fitted for wigs. I didn't recognize the person I had become when looking at in the mirror.

I was on a pain pump to try to find a tolerable pain level so I could go home. Being off the pain pump caused terrible withdrawal symptoms such as rolling around in bed at night screaming in pain to the point that I had to be sedated. I was living in a nightmare. My doctors finally found a tolerable pain medication in oral form that allowed me to go home. At one point, I was taking over 70 pills a day.

The following day, an IV port was placed in my chest before the ambulance took me back home. When I arrived back, my husband surprised me with family and close friends lined up along the driveway waiting to greet me, while waving encouraging signs. I felt so loved and happy to be back. My parents had a room ready for me with a lift chair. My two closest friends and my sister had a benefit planned for me. It touched my heart. The support and love from family and friends kept me going. I live in such a great community that rallied behind me. I was in a wheelchair and had to wear a bulky back brace that was uncomfortable with every move I made. I stayed at my local hospital for one week doing physical therapy and learning how to walk again. When I was discharged, my family and I moved in with my parents so they could help us. Home health came every week for routine blood work. Physical therapy came twice a week. I had countless doctor's appointments. Not only was I learning to walk again, I had to learn to go up and down steps. I could not dress myself. I felt the lowest of lows as I watched my husband and my parents sacrifice their time and energy to be my caretaker.

I had radiation on my back and hips along with the chemotherapy. The radiation caused two severe burns on my butt. I had to go to the wound clinic because they were so deep and painful. I was so sick. I vomited every day. I lost eighty pounds. I was miserable. I began to suffer from headaches. A brain MRI was ordered because of this. Tumors were found on my brain. Every day was a blessing and a struggle at the same time. I went straight back to Cleveland Clinic to have Gamma Knife radiation. Gamma Knife is a non-invasive medical procedure that uses precisely targeted gamma rays to treat certain brain conditions like tumors. It delivers focused radiation like a surgical knife, without an incision. Each spot took seventeen minutes to treat and over time I had over fifty tumors on my brain. My doctors told me I set the record for the most brain tumors at Cleveland Clinic.

Now, I visit Cleveland Clinic every three months for routine PET scans and brain MRIs. In June of 2022, I started an IV drug called Enhertu that I now get every three weeks at my local cancer center. I was the first person to ever start taking this infusion at my local cancer center.

Through all of this, I have never lost my faith or trust in God. I would blare my Christian music and cry out to Jesus begging Him to heal me so I could be here to watch my children grow up.

One evening, my mom and I visited a church that was having a night of worship. I fell in love with the atmosphere and it felt like home. I have always belonged to a church, however I knew this was where I wanted to be. Life Community Church provided me with a sense of comfort and a connection with God that has deepened over time. My pastor and my church family have played a crucial role in my journey toward a closer relationship with God. The power of prayer is remarkable in its ability to provide comfort, hope, healing and strength. My best friend's mother also took me to her church for blessings of healing and prayer as well.

My doctors were optimistic and told me that I would never be healed, however I know Jesus is my healer. In September of 2022, on my thirty-second birthday, I received the best gift yet. All of my scans were clear. I am living a miracle. All our prayers were answered. My doctors were amazing. My faith grew through healing. It has changed my heart and outlook on life. I have more of an appreciation for many things and am so blessed to be seeing my children grow up. I have met some of the greatest people along the way. I continue to fight and give my battles to God every day. Know your God! Never give up!

"I know someone who knows what I'm up against, I know someone who's here in the midst of it, fighting for me in a battle I can never win, all on my own!" "There is a power that is greater, so I'm not afraid of what's ahead - I'm standing in the confidence that even though I can't, my God can."

"My God Can," Katy Nichole featuring Naomi Raine

2 Kings 20:5 "I have heard your prayer and seen your tears; I will heal you."

ALL IN THE FAMILY

BY WANDA CLEAVER GEITNER

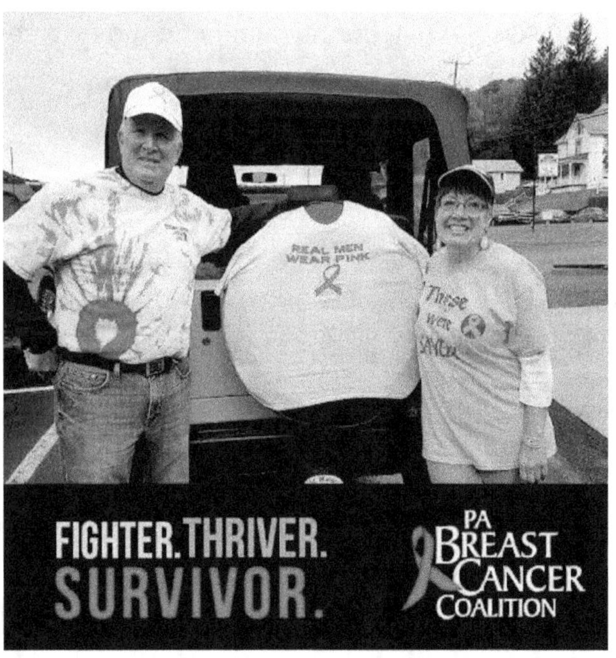

It was the summer of 2007. It was time for my annual mammogram, something I've been doing every year faithfully since I was in my early 30s because I was considered high risk for Breast Cancer. My mom, her two sisters (my aunts), and the majority of my cousins on my mother's side had all been diagnosed with breast cancer.

As I waited patiently in the room while the technician looked at my "pictures", she came from behind the screen and walked over and put her arms around my shoulders and gave me a hug and told me she found something. At that very moment, I felt as if she knew it was just not a normal insignificant lump. She showed me on the pictures and also helped me find it by placing my hand and moving my fingers exactly to the spot. I would have never found it if it wasn't for that mammogram! It was so very tiny.

Within the next hour they took me for a sonogram and my doctor was called. Oh, how I wished my mother was with me now. She had passed away 5 years earlier, not from the breast cancer that she endured 25 years earlier, but from heart failure.

I don't remember a lot about the next few days or couple of weeks. I do remember that at my biopsy the nurse came out to the waiting room and said that there was only a 1 in 10 chance that it would be breast cancer. I explained to her that I would be the 1 in 10 as so many women in my family had already been diagnosed, 2 of them passed away. My cousin

Sandy was only in her 50s and my cousin Denise lost her battle when she was only in her 30s.I was prepared!

When I went to see the Dr. for my results and he confirmed it was breast cancer, I was ready to have a complete mastectomy. I wanted it gone!! He explained to me that a lumpectomy was my best choice and I would have to possibly go through radiation and maybe chemo as well.

I went through the surgery, then a couple of months after recover, I began the chemo. The surgery was relatively easy and I had a quick recovery. The chemo made me sick but I did my best and made it through.

The radiation began a couple of months after my chemo had completed. I was able to work and function every day and drive myself for my treatments. I had 36 of them all together. The radiation was probably the worst of anything I went through. It burned my skin and they had to stop treatment for a few days. My insurance wouldn't pay for a "better" radiation treatment, as it was explained to me that if I had the "better" treatment I most likely wouldn't have gone through all the burning. My skin was literally peeling away. The pain was almost intolerable but I made it through, once again.

The entire process from the beginning of the diagnosis until I was totally finished was about a year. A very very long year. But here it is, 2024 and I am now a 17 year survivor! I have never had any problems or issues after everything.

At the time I was not married. I was living happily with my boyfriend. He was a Godsend through it all. We married in 2010.I don't know what I would've done without him by my side. Thank you JR for being my rock.

I always knew I would get breast cancer, but I also felt in my heart that I would not die from it!! I knew I would follow in my mother's footsteps and go on and live my life. I never ever take one single day for granted, as I know that can change in an instant.

The one and only cousin that did not have breast cancer when mine was discovered ended up with it a couple of years later. There isn't one woman in my mother's family that hasn't had breast cancer.

I had the genetic testing done because quite honestly I needed to for my families sake!! It was discovered that I did not have the BRCA gene. The doctors were shocked but also said that whatever genetic abnormality I had, it most likely had not been discovered yet.

This is just a condensed version of my life with breast cancer. I guess I have chosen to try to forget a lot of it; I no longer remember the entire medical part of it all...what exactly mine was, how I struggled with the day-to-day, etc. I am too busy living my life now.

Always, always get your mammograms faithfully. I am living proof of a reason why!! Without the early detection, I probably wouldn't be sitting here telling my story.

THE JOURNEY THAT NEVER ENDS

BY YVONNE CURLEY

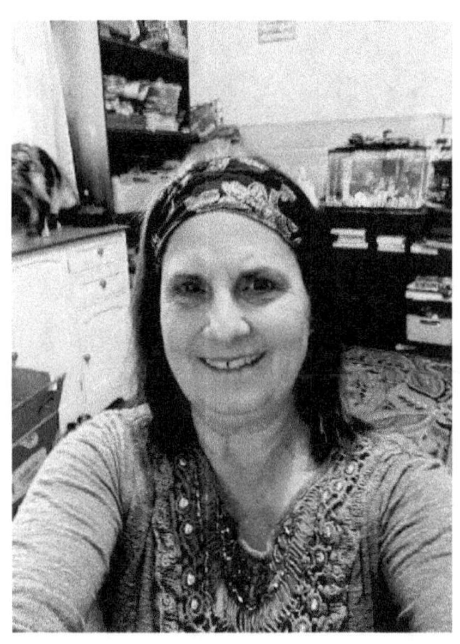

My cancer journey started over 20 years ago, in 2004. I became a warrior against Non-Hodgkin's Lymphoma. It is known as the "good cancer;" I don't know what is good about cancer, but ok. I guess it is because it is slow growing and it never truly goes away. The treatment was strong and rough, the side effects were awful. Chemo brain is a real thing, don't let anyone tell you differently! The biggest thing is they don't warn that the person you used to be is gone. The cancer and the chemo changes everything.

I did my treatments on Fridays so I could rest on the weekends. Mondays I was able to go back to work. I would sit for six hours hooked up to that lovely machine with the ice-cold medicine dripping slowly into my veins. I was thankful that I had faith and that God helped me through it. I would listen to Christian music and then fall asleep, six hours later it was all done, and I got to go home. Finally, I was done with Round 1.

In 2008, the war started again, tests and then treatment. I received 4 weekly doses of Rituximab, with one dose every six weeks for two years. Trying to stay involved is hard when you are afraid of catching anything and everything. Your immune system is so compromised during that time. Again, finally done with Round 2.

My childcare job was such a comfort to me, and I was so grateful to go to work. The children don't care if you are sick inside, they just want to love you no matter what, and I loved them. I think all those smiling faces and little people made me feel human again.

2012 here we went again, Round 3, ding ding, back in the ring I go. They found a mass behind my left eye. It was a low grade follicular lymphoma. More treatment and big adjustments. I was pretty much over it. From May to January 2014, I was DONE. I just didn't want to do it anymore. I cried all the time and I hurt all over. I couldn't sleep or remember certain things. I secluded myself, I felt so dumb saying or doing anything as I worked to find words and energy. People don't understand, they say you look fine. But it is on the inside that my whole world was falling apart. It was so bad that I even had someone say, "You are faking it; you look just fine, all you want is attention." I pray they are never in my shoes and have to learn the hard way.

I would pray, "God help me, I just want to be healthy again." Chemo changes you more mentally than physically. I started to change everything in my life; I made healthy choices, I was learning to accept one day at a time, I surrounded myself with my loving family and kept a positive attitude. I made plans for the future. It all seemed to be having a positive effect on me. I thought, "YAY, I am in remission!"

Nope.

In 2020 I had my routine scans, and I was feeling very optimistic. I was eating healthy, exercising, and taking care of my kiddos. However, my bubble burst with one phone call, "It's back". I reluctantly made a doctor's appointment to go over the results. I thought "Let's DO this, and get it OVER WITH." The biopsy showed Follicular Lymphoma, grade 1-2 B-cell. The testing began again, lots more tests, all uncomfortable and annoying. Thank God for the peace I did have through all the findings, which were not as bad as anticipated, but my bone scan detected a soft tissue hematoma in my left hip. No wonder it was so painful to walk, run, and play with the kids! I ended up having surgery to remove that mass.

I had to start treatment again. Every eight weeks I would go and receive Rituxan. I thought I was handling it pretty well; by January I had only a couple of treatments left to go. Jan 21, 2021, I got my treatment as usual, and I felt okay until I got home. I suddenly felt awful, and it just kept getting worse. I couldn't eat or drink anything at all. I wanted to just sleep all the time, I was so tired, I coughed all the time, when I tried to eat it tasted like metal or just horrible and I would spit it out because I couldn't even swallow it. I thought, I will drink more and try to keep hydrated. I couldn't do that either. I finally called the doctor. I was having an allergic reaction to the Rituxan. I started to lose a lot of weight; I was down to 104 lbs.! I felt like I was losing weight extremely fast! I forced myself to eat and drink; at least smoothies stayed down, and I could handle salads. I thought this was a sort of body cleanse and maybe it would help me feel better. It was working, after about 8 months I was finally feeling better.

Again, I was okay up until Dec 2023, when I had my routine scans. The results weren't good. A Pet scan was scheduled, and it made me so very sick. I got the worst headache and was throwing up. Never had this ever happened to me before. Then the results were in, the cancer was active again. They wanted me to go see a specialist in Pittsburgh PA at the Hillman Cancer Center. I was freaked out because I don't like to drive in Pittsburgh. Thank God for my friend Patty, she offered to take me. We had a nice trip and took the time to have a little fun while we were there (shopping at a second-hand store comes to mind). The good news was the visit went pretty well, as good as it could be! The cancer hadn't gotten any bigger or smaller, so we were able to start active surveillance and stop treatment.

In the meantime, I was told I needed my tonsils out, they were huge, and they needed to be removed and biopsied. This is a recent development, so at the time of this writing, I am still waiting for the results.

I know that God has a plan for me and it isn't up to me to understand what it is, I know in my heart He has something in store for me. My faith is strong and I will continue to trust in Him. My life is in His hands, and I know that I am not alone on the journey; I know He carries me. I am grateful for the life He has blessed me with, no matter how difficult at times.

CONTROL IS SUCH AN ILLUSION

BY CAIT WHITTLE THROOP

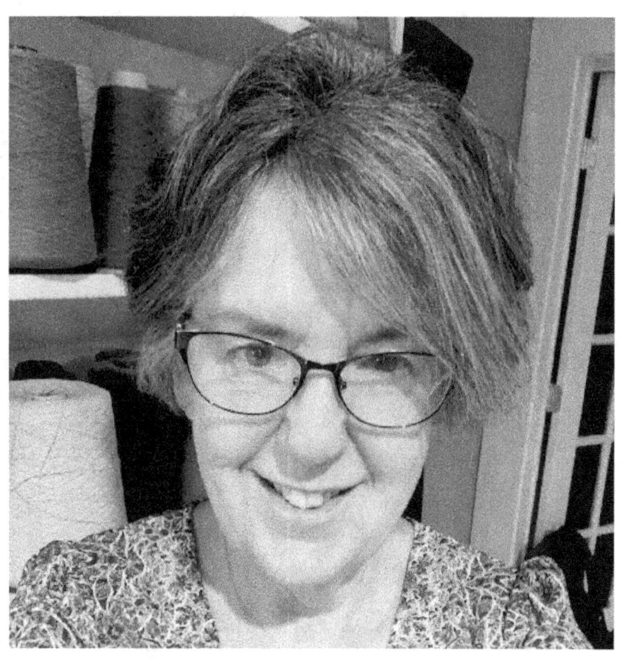

I turned 60 in May 2009, and within a couple of months something seemed wrong with my health. I was horse-back riding with a good friend, and I remember saying "I don't feel well. I don't feel sick but I don't feel well." In October I started itching. Itching in my hands and feet, so bad that I would scratch until they were bleeding. I didn't even have a doctor since having a hysterectomy at 48 so I went to urgent care. I was asked questions like; "Did you change detergents? I will give you a prescription for Benadryl" Although we didn't know it, we were so far beyond allergy meds. Finally, I found a nurse practitioner who prescribed a steroid. It didn't work, and by Thanksgiving I was sleeping (or trying to) with ice packs and finally I was staying up all night with my feet in ice water. The nurse practitioner sent me to Burlington, VT for an endoscopy. By that time, I was also jaundiced and very much wanting to give up. They found pancreatic cancer on December 13, 2009. Before I was fully awake the doctor told me I had pancreatic cancer. My only thought then was "what can we do about it?" My husband Gary, and my sister Eileen were told as I came out of surgery and as I woke up, they were already crying. I really didn't realize right then how serious it was. They were able to put in a stent so I felt much better, even if the situation was dire.

My husband and youngest son started research to find the best hospital to treat this. The more we found out the more shocking it was. All we could think was "how on earth can we deal with this?" Memorial Sloan Kettering in NYC was one of the top hospitals to do the Whipple surgery, so we went for an interview with the first doctor we saw on their list. Surgery was scheduled for January 6, 2010. My youngest turned 19 on January 5 and was with us. It was such a sad birthday, knowing the chances of survival were slim. The surgery and recovery, I have to say, were brutal. I went to my Mom's house in Keene, NH to recover so my husband could go back to work in northern NY. My youngest, Noah, and my middle son, Alex, tried taking me for a walk at JC Penney's to get some exercise. But I was losing weight rapidly because all food tasted like dirt in my mouth, and smells were absolutely horrible. I also had a fever so went to the Keene emergency room and they sent me by ambulance to NYC. That was an awful ride. I was readmitted to the hospital where they decided I was constipated. By this time, my oldest son, Adam, had arrived from Hawaii where he lived, and he and Noah kept me company. I was confused; could I be so badly constipated even though I hadn't eaten in a month by that time? The nurses lined up foul tasting liquid in little med cups on the tv tray and expected me to swallow them. I couldn't. Then came the enemas, which was a misery because I had a roommate who had male visitors when I had to get out of bed, cross the room "divided" by a curtain and get to the bathroom with med pole. This was totally ridiculous because as it turns out, I wasn't even constipated. Finally a lovely nurse told me I could refuse treatment which I did, and my sister Faith and husband rescued me and drove me back to my Mom's, where I slowly recovered.

By February I was home in northern NY but I was in so much pain and had a slight fever so I knew I had to go to the emergency room again. But first I took a shower! I knew if they did another surgery, it would be a while before I could wash my hair. Hey, some things are very important! This little country hospital knew immediately that I had a raging infection, so they reopened me and I had to heal by open stuffing the wound with gauze every day. That took some adjustment. By May I was healing but had lost 50 pounds. Chemo was relatively easy to deal with for 5 months and I was still alive, and happy to be here.

May 2016, I had an aortic valve replacement and in July while they were checking the results of that surgery with a CT scan, they saw what they thought was a scar on my right lung. In late December I had another CT scan and the scar had become a tumor. In January, while I was on the way down by bus for the women's march, I got a phone call from my thoracic nurse at 8 pm and she said that the doctor wanted to see me when I got back. Heads up; I had cancer again. In February 2017, it was back to Memorial Sloan Kettering to find a thoracic surgeon and schedule removing the top right lobe of my lung. This was robotically done, and it was the easiest of the surgeries with no chemo. However, we had to wait several months to find out what kind of cancer it was. Finally, I got a call from my original pancreatic surgeon and thought "Oh, this can't be good." He said it was pancreatic cancer to the lung. My thoracic surgeon was not as sure, so I still don't actually know if it was pancreatic or lung cancer.

In Spring 2019 I had a mammogram which showed a tumor after they saw something on the CT scan. I hadn't had a mammogram in years because I thought the CT scans covered everything and I was beginning to glow in the dark after so many scans. Silly, naïve me. My oncologist at the time never mentioned getting a mammogram so I thought everything was fine. Not so much. Again, on the right side. Several biopsies later, we were back in New York City and I had a lumpectomy for estrogen positive ductal carcinoma. And now instead of just the tumor being malignant, I had cancer in one of the lymph nodes as well. Then we started chemo. Nasty chemo, and radiation (which was easy). Then add in oral meds for at least 5 years. By this time, I had quite a list of doctors. I was supposed to self-check for lumps but because of the scarring and lumps from the lumpectomy and biopsies, physically I couldn't tell what was what.

In February 2021, a local surgeon thought she saw something on the CT scan so she did a biopsy which came back cancerous. Back to NYC to my breast surgeon. They did several biopsies but couldn't find anything. Finally, they got the original tissue from my local hospital and decided to do a mastectomy. But my heart valve wasn't doing a good job, so they wanted me to have another aortic valve replacement before I had breast surgery.

In the end of April 2021, we went back down to NYC to another hospital for heart surgery. It took until the fall to heal from that so it wasn't until October that I had the mastectomy. Recovery was tough from that one. First of all, I had a lot of swelling and had to be drained a couple of times. Second, I was somewhat depressed. I think the second breast cancer was the last straw. But anti-depressants came to the rescue as well as another lovely nurse practitioner who I could talk to and who listened and truly cared. That made all the difference. Now I have two shots every month on stronger anti-estrogen medications because obviously the oral medications didn't work. Fast forward to 2024 and the PET scan showed two lymph glands lit up on the chest wall. They can't biopsy because of the location so I will have a PET again in March to see if there are any changes.

The cancer timeline is one thing, but the emotional toll is another. My family has been there for me every step of the way. From figuring out the insurance crap to holding my hand and hugs when needed. In the hospital after the Whipple surgery, my kids came to see me, including my oldest who lives in Hawaii. When I got home my youngest had put lovely sayings all over the house. The one I remember most was inside a cupboard and said "When you are going through hell, keep on going." I am determined to use the time left to pursue what is important to me. My 3 sons, my two (soon to be 3) grandchildren, my art, my weaving, my horses, my friends. I have made it for my oldest son's wedding, and my middle son's wedding as well.

I have been going to a women's oncology camp almost every year since 2011 in the Adirondacks. I have met amazing, strong, inspiring women there. So much support and comradery, and just plain fun. For me, having cancer has driven it home how everyone's time here is getting shorter every day. So much for the Peter Pan complex. And how precious the time here is. And luckily I am not in any pain and can enjoy my life! I can't remember what the odds were for surviving pancreatic cancer, but I think I was told it was something like 7% over 5 years. My original surgeon told us that without surgery I would have a couple of months and with surgery maybe 2 years. It was so completely shocking. I still had so much to do. My youngest had just turned 19. I wanted to be here for them when they got married, had babies, whatever. That was a very difficult year.

Subsequent cancers have been easier to deal with although by the last breast cancer I was angry and sad and I had had enough. I think that once I recovered from each surgery, I felt okay and got my strength back so it made it easier to deal with. I haven't had any chronic pain which really does make a difference. My sister Faith has been there for me as well. She has been taking care of me while recovering, cooking meals, cleaning up, keeping me company. A friend comes every day to help with the horses. We heat our home with wood and when I came home from the hospital the first time, friends (anonymously) had filled the cellar with wood for heat that winter, all stacked and split. This thoughtful action truly brought me to tears. Friends have brought food, gifts, a listening ear, books, and love. There have been times in my life when I thought I had control. And I think my big life lesson is that control is such an illusion. However, I have learned that I am stronger than I ever thought I could be.

CAMP BRAVEHEARTS,

AN ONCOLOGY CAMP FOR WOMEN

Camp Bravehearts was established in 2001 after the three co-founders - Karen Haag, Lori Walsh and Joyce Chulock - attended a Women's Oncology Retreat weekend at "Camp Good Days and Special Times." in the Finger Lakes region of New York. Upon returning to Northeast Pennsylvania, they decided that similar retreats were needed in NEPA. The next year they branched out with headquarters in Albany, New York as well. Our all-volunteer leadership team keeps things flowing smoothly.

Camp Bravehearts is a non-profit organization that offers women dealing with any type of cancer a variety of weekend retreats, each focused on a different theme. Some retreats also provide opportunities to try the camper's skills at archery, kayaking, fishing, tackling a high ropes course, horseback riding, or hiking through majestic nature preserves. All participants can choose how much, if any, "adventuring" they would like to participate in. One concept remains the same, Camp Bravehearts is an experience of learning, healing, and sharing. We also provide several one-day programs that focus on wellness, healing and social events.

For those that would rather not be as adventurous, we offer crafts, silver jewelry making, swimming, wellness classes, games, and icebreakers, or just sitting in a gazebo reading a book or just chatting with other campers. One of the favorite activities is the annual Halloween costume party at the Double H Ranch in New York.

Our top priority is to serve women currently in treatment, women with metastatic and recurrent cancer, and newly diagnosed campers, which we have been doing for 23 years.

Here are a few of the many uplifting quotes from campers who have their lives enriched immensely by attending our weekend retreats.

"Oh my goodness, I cannot say enough about this experience. The people, the love, the space and the place! This first timer is hooked." Jolene

"Sitting here thinking about things, people, places, beautiful memories and my Bravehearts. Some of the memories bring me to tears thinking of dear friends I met at camp and missing them, but the majority of the memories bring a smile to my face and at times have me laughing! The love, encouragement and support was immediately thrown my way when arriving at camp." Christine

"I love coming to camp, it helps keep me in check, lets me know that I am not alone and I am grateful for having these opportunities." An anonymous Bravehearts camper.

"I am very grateful to be a part of Bravehearts. Cancer SUCKS! But the silver lining is that I have met the most amazing people at these retreats." An anonymous Bravehearts camper.

Tina

To find out more go to:

https://braveheartscamp.org/

Or check out the Facebook Page:

https://www.facebook.com/groups/320764192272

The Double H Ranch, co-founded by Charles R. Wood and Paul Newman, provides specialized programs and year-round support for children and their families dealing with life-threatening illnesses. Our purpose is to enrich their lives and provide camp experiences that are memorable, exciting, fun, empowering, physically safe and medically sound. All programs are FREE of charge and capture the magic of the Adirondacks!

In the Spring and Fall we host an organization, Camp Bravehearts, which is for women in treatment for cancer or who have had cancer. The ladies that attend Camp Bravehearts are some of the most inspiring people I have ever met. They celebrate life, lift each other up and hold space for each other to listen and be present.

Whether during Camp Bravehearts or our traditional camp programming, Double H Ranch is a refuge for families, a home away from home for our campers and a garden where everyone involved is the best version of themselves and all flourish mutually. Challenges are met, new friends are made, lessons are learned, and smiles and laughter abound.

-Health & Happiness

Chris Pezzulo

For more information on The Double H Ranch check out the website:

https://www.doublehranch.org/

Facebook page also:

https://www.facebook.com/DoubleHRanchCamp

ENDING THOUGHTS:

I was 51 when I was first diagnosed with cancer. As the mother to 2 adult children, the wife to an amazing husband (as of this writing) of 36 years, and as the daughter/caregiver to disabled parents, the emotional hit drove me to my knees. Like every woman, how could I juggle cancer along with everything I was already doing? I had a demanding but incredibly enjoyable career as a Speech Language Pathologist, and I had just entered the competitive world of private practice. How could I continue to work to my level, exploding with fun, laughter and support for my clients? Where would I find the strength?

Treatment started, and the exhaustion was MASSIVE. We had recently moved to a beach community on the North Shore of Long Island, so I gave myself the task of walking the beaches. I knew that sitting home would be the wrong decision; I needed to move, and being out in nature has always been healing for me. I would order myself; "Go for a walk." As I walked and looked at the rocks, I added a new task: "Pick up and collect beach glass." What I was going to do with it, I didn't know, but it felt right.

Over the past 7 years, I have collected thousands of pieces of beach glass. Each one was different; each one showed its scars of being thrown about in Long Island Sound. I did some crafts, gave some to crafty friends, and sorted the pieces by size/color/shape. However, what I really loved to do was just hold it, run my thumbs over it, and absorb the changes.

What makes beach glass different from other glass? Beach glass is formed when broken, discarded glass is tumbled by waves continuously, while the sharp edges dull and the glass itself absorbs minerals from the water. After many years, the glass that is left resembles a rock; it is no longer translucent, there are no sharp edges, and the glass is cloudy. One other change; the glass is STRONG. The glass is strengthened by the minerals it absorbs.

The parallels between cancer and beach glass were clear to me (pardon the pun). Cancer breaks us, turns us into sharp shards that take a long time to dull. At the same time, while we are being tossed about, if we can keep from breaking, we absorb what we need to make us stronger.

As I somehow came to accept my uncertain future, I decided to explore options for engaging in a cancer retreat. I found Bravehearts, and the love, humor, and support I found there was truly healing. And every woman I met had absorbed what she needed to strengthen herself against that which should have broken her. For some it was religion, for others it was meditation, other need nature; there is no one answer for everyone. However, there is an answer for everyone.

Please find your peace; please find what strengthens you against the rushing waters of Life.

~Nancy

I APPLAUDED ALL OF YOU

Wow, what a humbling experience this has been. I found myself in tears many nights reading these stories. So many of these stories seem to come alive right before my eyes as I could feel and see what was going on with each one of the writers.

Isn't the power of the human spirit amazing? How we dig deep and find that inner strength to rise above, to keep moving forward.

I hope these stories have inspired you. As I was told a long time ago, we take what we need and we leave the rest. I am hoping you found what you needed in these stories.

I know it has renewed my faith in the human spirit. I also found that a common thread in many of these stories was their faith in God/ higher spirit. We do not always like to admit it, but we can't do any of this alone. I have been shown too many times that I am not alone.

I personally want to "Thank you" for taking the time to read these stories. I hope you understand how hard it was for some of them to open up a very private battle they had in their lives and share it with the world. I am so glad they did!

If you are struggling right now with something going on in your life, know there is hope and never give up. Just take it as it comes and look ahead for tomorrow. We are all here to help each other along the way. Be kind to yourself and be kind to others. You never know what is going on in their world.

I really want to thank Nancy Stein for jumping right in to help me with editing and helping me through some rough spots. She has been a blessing! Who would have thought that my bunk buddy and I would be doing this a year later! Aww… there is no coincidence is there. You just never know who God puts in your path huh?

If you would like to donate to Braveheart here is the address:

Camp Bravehearts, Inc.
19 Cambridge Road
Albany, NY 12203

If you would like to donate to The Double H Ranch:

DOUBLE H RANCH | A SERIOUSFUN CAMP
97 Hidden Valley Road, Lake Luzerne, NY 12846

If you have a story you would like to share, I would love to hear from you, please drop me a line.

Patricia Greene
elkcounty2020@gmail.com

Check out my other books on Amazon:

Ripples: Effects of Addiction
Ripples: Stories of Addiction: Recovery is Possible

Patricia Greene